My Life Well-Adjusted

A Life Worth Living

Dr. Jeffrey Slocum

My Life Well-Adjusted
Copyright © 2018 by Jeffrey Slocum
Printed and bound in the United States.

First printing July, 2018

Table of Contents

Dedication

This book would not be possible if it weren't for the love and understanding of my tirelessly supportive wife Debbie. Debbie has patiently allowed me to follow my passion for the practice of chiropractic, my quest to become an effective leader, and my drive to serve my community. I have been blessed to be able to dedicate much of my professional life knowing she is anchoring my personal life, including raising our 3 amazing children.

Another unwavering and unshakable pillar of support in my life for the past 15 years is my colleague, partner, mentor, and most importantly, my dear friend Dr. Rok Morin. I am where I am today because of the influence that Debbie and Rok have had on my life personally and professionally.

I'm grateful for the relationship I've had with my professional coach and good friend Dr. Alan Rousso, who has helped shape my vision, challenged me to grow, given me a hand when I failed, and has always been there to celebrate my accomplishments.

I'd also like to acknowledge the other partners, Dr. Jeremy Book, Dr. Tim Coffin, and Dr. Mike Epperson, and our teams of dedicated doctors and para-professionals at the Chiropractic Vitality Centers of Maine. They make it all happen!

I never would have pursued the practice of full-scope chiropractic or developed the "My Life Well-Adjusted" model if it were not for the 10 family members who practiced before me. I am especially and eternally grateful for the wisdom of my grandfather, Dr. William Smith, my first "job" as an associate with my father, Dr. Roy Slocum, and my oldest brother and chiropractic college roommate, Dr. Dustin Slocum. They set the stage for my early career and inspired me to always work at honing my skills.

Thank you to my assistant, proof reader, biggest fan, and most importantly MOM, Jenene Slocum for making my life manageable!

Lastly, I dedicate this book to my incredible children Isabella, Amelia, and Andrew for whom I am simply "dad." Being your father is the most important job I will ever have, and it is the best job I could ever ask for!

I am thankful and humbled by the contributions you've all made to my life, and I am glad to share this book with you, as it couldn't have happened without you.

Foreword

For the last 17 years I have had a front row seat to the evolution of Dr. Jeffrey Slocum. Like many things in life it was a strange turn of events that brought us together, but it happened at the perfect time for both of us, as we were going through personal challenges in our lives. Through that process we grew an incredible practice that served many people in our community, developed an incredible partnership, but most of all formed an amazing friendship. It is my honor to be able to write this introduction for Dr. Slocum's first book

As I said, I have had a front row seat to the changes in Dr. Slocum's life. I have seen him change practices as we expanded our influence around Maine. I have seen him evolve as a chiropractor as changes in techniques, technology and insurance have changed around us. Most importantly, I have seen Dr. Slocum do the hard work to change himself to become the best version of himself he can possibly be.

This book is the culmination of growing up in a chiropractic family and practicing chiropractic for 25 years, taking care of and coaching thousands of people. It is also drawn from his own journey of personal discovery, health and wellness. The concepts of living a healthy lifestyle are simple. It's the practice and application that are difficult. This book is a tool to be used to help you on your journey.

One thing that hasn't changed over all these years is Dr. Slocum's desire to help people and the excitement he gets when he sees other people achieving their goals.
Personally, I would not be where I am today without my relationship with my friend Jeff. Take this book, apply the principles outlined, enjoy the great benefits, and repeat for as long as you want to continue to grow and prosper.

God Bless,

Dr. Rok A. Morin

Chapter 1

My Life Well-Adjusted

By digging into this book, you're about to take a journey of imagination, hard work and empowered living. I want to encourage you to use this book as a catalyst to begin your personal life journey with your optimal goals as a desired outcome. It's my hope that when you're finished reading the last page, you'll have a clear and undeniable understanding of what "My Life Well-Adjusted" is all about!

Whether you use "My Life Well-Adjusted" as a course in self-study, or you allow me to facilitate and coach you through this creative and rewarding adventure, my intention is to help you create *A Life Worth Living*. When I say that, I don't mean to sound trite or judgmental. I intend it to be inspirational, to create an atmosphere of hopeful imagination that will lead to a state of self-determined certainty, and that will guide you to build the life you desire most: a life that is fantastically meaningful and fulfilling!

Time allows for clarity and wisdom. When we seek the clarity and wisdom of the people who've come before us we can learn and use the lessons they've gleaned from experience and life reflection. When asked later in their lives, many people admit that life is most often directed and guided by chance, not by definition. Very few people experience a life directed by laser-like consciousness that is defined by the forethought or designed out of clarity of values, vision, and purpose.

"My Life Well-Adjusted" is designed to offer the possibility of greater consciousness, a more focused development of empowered ideas and concepts, a well-defined and disciplined lifestyle, and purposeful actions that will lead you to the outcome of a truly meaningful life experience.

In the "My Life Well-Adjusted" journey, there are 2 separate but inseparable tracks that are worked on simultaneously:

Track 1: Physical and Physiological Well-Being
(Full-Scope Chiropractic for Structural, Neurological, and Physiological Adaptability)

Track 2: Whole Life Planning and Development
(7 Dimensions of Life with the Success Triad)

Building a well-adjusted life is about becoming very clear on who you are, what you want to accomplish, learning how to purposefully pursue your life with a higher level of conscious planning, and having the physiological health necessary to enjoy it to the fullest. The design and implementation of the "My Life Well-Adjusted" program was born from the accumulated years of studying success systems, the lessons I've learned from many mistakes and many celebrated victories, as well as listening to and learning from people who have achieved the level of success and fulfillment that I desired to emulate.

Some of the lessons that I teach in the "My Life Well-Adjusted" program have been harvested from the experiences I had with the adults who shaped my childhood years, and what I've learned as a parent raising 3 amazing children. Other aspects of the "My Life Well-Adjusted" program are a direct reflection of the growth I've experienced while working with colleagues and coaches in my professional life, or what I've learned about life from people of influence, and the interactions I've had the honor to develop through leadership roles in my practice communities.

Lastly, the work I do with my clients is deeply rooted in the skill sets I've accumulated in my 25 years of professional practice as a care provider, coach, boss, and partner with the doctors and teams of the Chiropractic Vitality Center of Maine.

In this book, I'll introduce you to a model of business success originally developed as a consulting model for professionals called "Advanced Leadership Solutions." The reason I've adapted it to my chiropractic practice is simple: when we looked at the totality of the experience of our original professional "graduates," we saw the results bled into the much broader arena of private life for many.

When I looked at the results of our professional clients and assessed what I felt was missing in the experience of my chiropractic practice members, I realized that life planning and development was the missing ingredient. In the "My Life Well-Adjusted" model, we've changed the focus of the previous professional model to a more inclusive life model and named it more aptly: "The Success Triad." True health is a multidimensional state, and the "My Life Well-Adjusted" program has allowed us to help our clients develop a multidimensional wellness outcome.

"My Life Well-Adjusted" uses the design of the Success Triad: **Be Genuine, See Clearly, Act Purposefully**.

The Success Triad can guide you through the process of defining, with certainty, who you are and what makes you tick, from a core values standpoint. This, in effect, allows you to **Be Genuine**.

To **Be Genuine** is to be fully aware of your core values. Your core values are the fuel and/or catalyst that drives you. In fact, your core values are the bedrock of your personal character. They are the brick and mortar of the why, what, and how of your life.

Becoming fully conscious of your core values adds a layer of consciousness that allows you to maximize your effectiveness and minimize your effort. Understanding who you are is critical to helping you determine what you really want. When is the last time you took a reasonable amount of time to get completely clear on what you really wanted?

Investing your energy and attention in the "My Life Well-Adjusted" process will direct your drive and crystalize your desire to determine, with clarity, what you want to accomplish with the time you have to live this life, and WHY you want to accomplish it.

To **See Clearly** is to be able to define what you want to accomplish and have a vision of the outcome that is crystal clear and compelling enough to build the desire to work for it with discipline and perseverance. How great do you think it will feel to be able to **See Clearly** a vision of your life as you define and design it? What if there were no rules and you could set and achieve your goals? Not wishes, but real tangible goals with less effort and greater success? Wouldn't it be nice to be able to become more aware, more certain, and more defined in the design of your ideal life?

The third aspect of the Success Triad is the deployment of your core values in the direction of your defined vision, which allows you to **Act Purposefully** in 7 dimensions of life. In moments of awareness, having your core values and your vision written in proverbial stone will allow you to immediately assess whether to move on with no emotional connection or to **Act Purposefully.**

You're not alone if you've ever found yourself aware of a situation that needed attention but were unsure of whether to let it go (as it may not really have mattered), or to act (because it was important to your purpose in life). I call these the moments of "awkward awareness," and life is full of these moments!

Awkward awareness moments are often a reflection of uncertainty or possibly even a question of values or vision clarity. There is good news: once you've done the foundational work of the values assessment and learn to **Be Genuine**, the vision development so you can **See Clearly**, and you have the capacity to move forward and **Act Purposefully**, those awkward awareness moments will go away, become less frequent, and completely disappear in some dimensions of life!

As a final activity of the Success Triad, define, design, and deploy model of "My Life Well-Adjusted," you'll work with the "process to purpose" clarity tool for the 7 dimensions of your life that are most definable and actionable.

These dimensions (in no particular order of importance) are physical, mental, social, financial, spiritual, professional, and emotional. I say no order of importance, but there does seem to be an order that is most productive. I generally recommend with most clients that we begin with the physical and physiological dimensions, as these are the 2 dimensions of life that we are most comfortable and conscious of, and lead to BIG success right out of the gate!

The process is different for each client, and in the end, regardless of where we start first, when we work on any dimension of life we effect all dimensions of life. It's as JFK stated in his famous quote, "A rising tide lifts all boats."

If this sounds like a desired state for you, I'm here to tell you it's not only possible, it's probable, if you invest in yourself and decide to do the work required to **Be Genuine, See Clearly, and Act Purposefully**.

"It's better to be a meaningful specific than a wandering generality."

I'm really excited to take this journey with you, and I hope that you'll engage with hopeful optimism and an unrelenting imagination of what can come to be for your life well-adjusted. From my experience in practice, as a coach and a mentor to colleagues, as a leader in my corporate work, as a parent, and as a human going along my life path to this point, I can tell you that the option to do "whatever" and just go with the flow seldom leads to the mountain top.

In the quiet moments of reflection at the end of a career or life, you don't hear many people say they wished they'd spent more time at the office, had taken fewer vacations, had saved less money, had planned less for retirement, had given more to their work, or waited longer to get healthy. Those are not the wishes of most people in their moments of life reflection!

In the quiet moments at the end of life, more people wish they had more meaningful and specific goals, had focused more energy and attention to the most importance areas of their life, had acted earlier on their dreams, had started taking better care of their health earlier, had saved more money or taken more vacations, had taken more time to appreciate the finer aspects of life, and finally, had spent more time with the people who made their lives whole in the places that inspire them.

"My Life Well-Adjusted" is an inspired process designed to help you create the most well-rounded, balanced, structured, purposeful, vision-based, goal-oriented, rewarding, confident, and meaningful life possible.

"My Life Well-Adjusted," by design, is a comprehensive, 52-week journey of discovery and growth designed with the specific intention to help you achieve the core aspects of being well. There is no aspect of the work of "My Life Well-Adjusted" by itself that would fail to have a meaningful impact on your life if done separately. To realize the maximum impact of the totality of the "My Life Well-Adjusted" journey, I recommend that it be tackled with a determined hopefulness and full engagement.

I would not suggest that my years or style of practice was deficient in any way, as I've been able to help a lot of people regain and maintain a level of health which they failed to achieve before we worked together. More accurately, or specifically, I would say that I personally and professionally have been called to practice a more "whole life inclusive" style of care program that fits my professional desire more fully at this stage of my career. I'm glad I listened to that (not so quiet) voice inside my head as it called me to develop and coach the advanced "My Life Well-Adjusted" program.

Structure Dictates Function

If you decide to fully engage and work with me or one of our "My Life Well-Adjusted" doctors, you will undergo a comprehensive spinal, neurological, physiological program of care throughout the full 52-week program known as "Track 1." Track 1 of "My Life Well-Adjusted" starts on day one and continues through 3 phases of full-scope care throughout the journey. The focus on spinal, neurological, and physiological balance is to maximize your innate ability to self-heal, self-regulate, control and coordinate your internal environment, and ensure full adaptation to life stresses in your external environment. The chiropractic component of "My Life Well-Adjusted" will set the physical and physiological framework to support the life adjustment and ensures that the whole journey creates optimal well-being and the full expression of health in 7 dimensions of life.

Tracks of the "My Life Well-Adjusted" program

Track 1: Physical and Physiological Well-Being

Acute Phase

In this first phase of care, the main goal is to correct spinal instability (called a *vertebral subluxation complex*) and the resulting nerve interference, which is the cause of physiological imbalance, reduced health expression, and limited adaptability. Often there is a rapid reduction of symptoms in the acute phase, but the healing of the underlying cause is just starting. Restoration of the natural healing potential of the body in the acute phase requires frequent visits over a short duration of time. The frequency and duration of acute care is determined by the objective findings of your exam, the goals you have for your future health, and the ability your body has to heal.

Most people are under the assumption that if they don't feel any pain then there is nothing wrong with them, and they're "healthy." Unfortunately, pain is a very poor indicator of health. In fact, pain and other symptoms frequently only appear after a disease process has gone undetected and uncorrected for a prolonged period of time.

All care in a full-scope chiropractic model is directed to address objective measurements of disease and bring the healing potential of the body back to balance. Most chiropractors regard the elimination of symptoms as the easiest part of a person's care. If all a chiropractor does is reduce pain and stop there, the chances of the cause of your condition recurring and becoming much more devastating is a guarantee! It's not the goal of health care to reduce symptoms, but to restore health. Fortunately, symptoms tend to go away as health expression returns.

Rehabilitative Phase

The Rehabilitative phase of full-scope chiropractic care is purposefully designed to facilitate a more robust and complete healing process, structurally, neurologically, cellularly, and physiologically. There are specialized nerve fibers that live in and around your joints that are responsible for sending messages to the brain and from the brain to the body. These nerves and the quality and quantity of the information they carry are what help your body self-regulate and heal efficiently and effectively.

This phase of care goes well beyond your initial subjective complaint and focuses on your body's healing potential, thus affecting all systems and cellular functions, and will ultimately set the stage for the return of a more complete health expression. During the rehabilitative phase of care, you'll receive less frequent adjustments due to the fact that your body is better able to heal, self-regulate, and adapt to the normal stresses of life again. Rehabilitative care is generally a longer and more impactful phase of care, as we are setting the stage for the "grand finale" of health care called wellness care.

Wellness Phase

The wellness phase of care is true "health care" versus what most people think of in the world of symptom based "sick care." Wellness starts when your body is able to adapt to stress in the physical, chemical, and mental/emotional realms of life. Once your body has fully healed, regular chiropractic care will help ensure that you maintain proper spinal and neurological balance, so you can trust your body and enjoy a full and active life of optimal health expression.

Proper spinal care in a wellness model is similar to any other aspect of a healthy life, like exercise, diet, hydration, or rest, in that it's necessary to prevent injury or disease at a minimum, and to facilitate full health expression as a premier outcome.

This phase of care is where you'll learn to appreciate how important your spinal health is to your total health! You'll truly understand and fully experience how maintaining a balanced spine creates abundant health and greater freedom from sickness. Wellness care has the lowest frequency of care, but the duration is for life if you choose to make a healthy spinal system a priority.

Track 2: Whole Life Planning and Development

Be Genuine

In the first step of the whole life planning and development track we will work with you to complete the values assessment portion of "My Life Well-Adjusted." This isn't a rushed process, and it will take several working sessions with your coach. Defining and designing your optimal life is an in-depth and powerful initial set point for your future, and it deserves as much time as it takes. In the values assessment, you define the primary core values that allow you to move from awareness to action, with clarity, certainty and confidence. The values assessment will help you define the secondary values that support your core values as you bridge the gap between awareness and purposeful action.

To lend clarity of concept, consider awareness and action to be 2 mountains separated by a valley. The valley is where "awkward awareness" lives. It's where fear, doubt, uncertainty, and procrastination live. When you have your core and secondary values securely acknowledged, you can move from awareness to action using the values bridge of certainty and avoid the valley of dreaded uncertainty. During this process, there is homework assigned and reading to be completed so that the foundational consciousness is developed, and the first stage of the Success Triad is built.

See Clearly

In the second step of the whole life planning and development track, the focus is on the creation of the vision you have for the 7 key dimensions of your life. In this phase, we'll focus on building clearly defined, inspired, and meaningful goals that are consistent with your core values, align with your vision, and set the stage for the future you desire.

In the **See Clearly** phase of the whole life planning and development track, you'll become aware that many of the habitual reactions you currently have in daily life are not truly purposeful as defined by your core values. You may also come to realize that much of your energy is spent reacting to a demand of time, money, energy, and resources, or simply done without a tremendous amount of conscious forethought, emotionally balanced energy, or directed at well-defined goals.

At the end of the **See Clearly** phase of the whole life planning and development track, you'll have clear and compelling goals, with a crystallized vision that most people never take the initiative to develop. You'll have a life compass which will guide you in your actions and ensure you are more purposefully engaged in the pursuit of your destiny.

Act Purposefully

The third stage of the whole life planning and development track is designed to use our "process to purpose clarity tool" to develop a sound and stable values statement as it pertains to critically areas of the 7 dimensions of your ideal life. This will be your "mission" statement if you will, and it will guide your actions in key areas that are fundamental to the attainment of the vision of life you desire to create. When we have a values statement to fuel our actions and vision statement to direct our efforts, we can **Act Purposefully**.

Purposeful action is action that aligns with our values and vision, any action that does not align in this way wastes time, energy, and valuable resources.

Putting it all together

The "My Life Well-Adjusted" journey has a starting point, but no end. This whole life adjustment plan is the first 52 weeks of the rest of your well-defined life journey. It's my goal that by the end of the year, you will possess the skills, the knowledge, and the certainty to integrate the Success Triad into your life.

If you take advantage of the full-scope of the "My Life Well-Adjusted" program and give it everything you have, you'll have a new consciousness that you can apply to real-life scenarios that affect your multidimensional life. You'll see more often that there is new meaning and more fulfillment in your daily life, and it will show up as the successful achievement of measurable goals!

When you're able to **Be Genuine, See Clearly, and Act Purposefully**, you will bridge the gap from awareness to action with ease and confidence.

Warning

There is one very important distinction that must be made up front which is essential to your full experience and long-term success: *You will do the work. We do not do the work for you.*

We will coach, guide, challenge, support, and facilitate your journey of discovery, but this is your growth experience, designed by us and defined by you. Success comes from the ability to move from awareness to action with certainty, confidence and high self-esteem. This journey and the experience and expansion you create will be yours forever, and we desire to make sure that it creates extreme value in helping you create your well-adjusted life, and *A Life Worth Living*!

I have the distinct honor and pride of celebrating my 25th year of chiropractic practice as of the writing of this book, and I owe a level of gratitude beyond expression to those who've shaped me personally and professionally. I'm very fortunate to be the 11th chiropractor spanning 4 generations in my family, as well as having had the good fortune to have worked with the partners of The Chiropractic Vitality Centers of Maine, in service to literally tens of thousands of individuals and families!

You'll see through this book and/or through the work we do together (if I'm fortunate enough to earn your trust), that I am fully invested in a powerful truth: a focus on spinal integrity and neurological adaptability must be the starting point for creating optimal wellness in your life.

Through my personal experience and my professional practice, I understand this inherent truth so completely, that I've committed the next 2 chapters to explain in detail the direct and undeniable relationship between the spine, the nervous system, and your health expression.

Every high achiever on this planet who is at the top of their game has a coach! If you simply choose to read this book as a self-study guide, I truly hope you enjoy the clarity it creates and the results you achieve. If, however, you decide to work with me to coach, guide, and care for you through the meaningful and exciting journey of creating your well-adjusted life, I would be honored! I'm extremely excited to share this journey with you and would relish the opportunity to see you succeed and/or hear your feedback!

If you are ready to start the "My Life Well-Adjusted" journey, contact Dr. Jeffrey Slocum today.

Dr. Jeffrey Slocum, owner of Bangor Family Chiropractic and developer and head coach at My Life Well-Adjusted
207-307-7513 ● drjeff@mylifewelladjusted.com

Chapter 2

You Live Your Life through your Nervous System

"The foundation of living a well-adjusted life starts with understanding and empowerment."

- Jeffrey Slocum, D.C.

To develop the understanding required to optimize your well-adjusted life, it's essential that we begin at the core of "life." The core premise of living a well-adjusted or optimized life is to understand this powerful concept: *the nervous system is the master system of your body.*

The nervous system is the control module for healthy adaptability, self-regulation, systems control, and physiological balance. In modern vernacular, it's appropriate to think of the central and peripheral nervous systems as the software that runs your life. Later in this chapter, and deeper into your journey through the "My Life Well-Adjusted" experience, I'll explain how the spinal system (the hardware) houses and supports the nervous system (the software) and is inseparable in its importance to neurological adaptability and full health expression.

The central nervous system as we will discuss it here is made up of 2 distinct parts:

1) The central nervous system, being the brain and the spinal cord that runs through the spinal column.

2) The peripheral nervous system, being all the nerve bundles and cells that branch off the spinal cord and exit through the spinal column, to regulate directly or indirectly every cell, tissue, and organ in the body.

The nervous system as a whole is without a doubt the primary or master system of the body, not just theoretically, but literally. The central and peripheral nervous systems control, coordinate, and regulate every action, reaction, and system, including:

- Digestion
- Assimilation
- Muscle (motor) control
- Temperature regulation
- Immune responses
- Cellular growth
- Respiration
- Blood pressure
- Balance
- Mobility
- Memory
- Emotion
- You name it!

From the instant you were conceived to this moment reading this chapter, your nervous system has been at the helm of your life experience. It's shaped every aspect of your life, including the physical, chemical, emotional, and intellectual. In fact, the nervous system is so deeply connected to "who you are," it was the first tissue that developed in utero. All other cellular growth and coordination of cellular organization, including the development of the spinal column, stems from the initial structure called the notochord.

The nervous system and all your sensory organs allow you to understand your environment, both external and internal, coordinate biological function, react and respond to ALL challenges or stresses, whether they be physical, chemical, and/or mental/emotional and to coordinate the efforts of all systems to work together in harmony and balance. The saying, "you live your life through your nervous system" is not just a slogan, it's the absolute truth.

In thousands of instances in my private practice I've found that once one understands and honors the locus of control within the body, one begins to recognize and seek ways to support one's own magnificent nervous system. There are specific lifestyle choices that increase your adaptive potential, so you can express greater health and minimize the development of disease.

Understanding the role of the spinal system and the nervous system in the development of healthy adaptation will empower your thoughts, actions, and outcomes, and help you navigate the physical, chemical, and mental/emotional stresses we call life. Knowledge is power, and with this knowledge you can tip the balance of life in your favor by understanding how health and sickness occur.

Learning the relationship between structural integrity and neural adaptability is, in my opinion, the most important aspect of health we should learn as we develop our world view. Sadly, most people never hear the truth until it's too late. Once you know the relationship (which you will when you complete this book) you will understand the inherent need to maintain a flexible and functional spinal system as it relates to the full expression of health, through proper and full neurological control and communication, from above down and inside out (ADIO).

Your nervous system functions as an input/output loop, constantly taking into account all internal needs and external stressors as it balances the 2 opposite forces in homeostasis. With my practice members and with the audiences in my community, I explain the result of inputs and outputs in this very simple way: good inputs lead to good outcomes, bad inputs lead to bad outcomes. The body, as a result of the relationship between structure and function, is either in a state of adaptation called ease which is healthy, vital, and natural, or it is in a state of compensation called dis-ease which is unhealthy, destructive, and unnatural.

The natural and normal state of the body is one of ease, which is a state of balance or homeostasis, where the brain and the body are communicating. The body can self-regulate, it can adapt to stressful inputs in healthy ways, and it's capable of coordinating all the systems in balance and harmony. In a state of ease, the brain and body communicate messages in a constant, uninterrupted feedback loop. In this state of ease the message is clear, concise, and understandable, the action is pure, and the outcome is desirable and optimized.

This messaging happens literally billions of times per second in the human body, and ultimately shapes your health and your total experience in life. When your body is balanced structurally and neurologically, you've achieved a state of ease, or homeostasis. You might sense ease as an optimal expression of health beyond just how you feel, but more importantly, how you function.

The unnatural and abnormal state of the body is one of dis-ease, which is a state of imbalance, where the brain and body do not communicate fully or harmoniously. When the body is out of balance or homeostasis, there's a lack of self-regulation and system coordination, which causes an immediate loss of neurological adaptability and dis-ease. You might sense dis-ease as a less than optimal expression of health and vitality. When dis-ease is left undetected and uncorrected in the body, it eventually shows up as a full-blown disease process.

Even though a diagnosis of diabetes, arthritis, heart disease, or cancer can seem like it comes out of left field, there's no such thing as a freak occurrence in the body. Every health expression or expression of sickness is a process that has occurred through inputs and outcomes over time. We don't become "sick" in the moment the signs and symptoms of disease show up, we become "sick" as soon as we develop dis-ease.

The symptoms that eventually appear are a result of the body's lack of adaptability to stress and its inability to coordinate health. Symptoms are the end stage of dis-ease, not the cause of it, and therefore the development of symptoms is necessarily a process of time. Symptoms are often the last thing that shows up.

Consider the example of a dental cavity, for instance. A cavity is caused by bacteria that eats through the enamel, and over time makes its way through the pulp of a tooth until it finally hits the nerve root, and that's when the symptoms show up. Just as in the example of dental disease, most diseases start long before the first symptoms show up. This is true for all the major diseases you've heard of, or possibly even have experienced first-hand, such as heart disease, cancer, diabetes, spinal disease (arthritis), and so on.

To help understand how the spinal system affects neurological function, and therefore physiology, I'll state again that the spinal column is the house (hardware) of the central nervous system and its protective outer cover. This doesn't even begin to explain the deep and indivisible relationship between the spine and the nervous system, but it's a starting point.

If there's a need to build a deeper case to bolster the evidence for the importance of the spinal column, we only need to look to the fact that our nervous system is the only tissue or organ in the body that has a protective covering. The brain has the skull to protect and house it, and the spinal cord has the spinal column to provide anchoring points for its outer lining, and to provide the perfect shape, length, and structure to ensure its safety.

The spinal column is also supremely important to the nervous system as a conduit to carry the spinal cord, and as the perfect vessel to provide the space and spacing necessary to off-shoot peripheral nerves to innervate all tissues of the body. Without a balanced, flexible, and structurally sound spinal column there would be no way for the brain and body to communicate, or to allow for the harmonious input /output messaging feedback loop that allows for the optimal expression of health through adaptability.

The reasons we have a spinal column are many, including flexibility to accommodate our active lives, weight bearing strength and adaptation to gravity, and anchoring points of many postural and skeletal muscles. However, the biggest reason we have a spinal column is simple: if the nervous system had no home, it would be impossible for the brain and the body to communicate back and forth, and we'd be unable to survive, let alone to thrive.

In the next chapter, I'll go into a detailed explanation of the mechanism by which the joints in our spinal column and our axial skeleton affect brain function and neurological adaptation. For now, let's leave it at this: the spinal column as it's designed is both a mechanical and a neurological structure, as well as a sensor and a sender of neurological information between the brain, the body, and the internal and external environments that affect our overall health.

There are specialized nerve fibers that are essential for self-regulation and systems control, which are most highly concentrated in our spinal tissues, but they're also present in our muscles, ligaments, tendons, discs, cartilage, skin, and other soft tissue in our body. As our spinal column moves, flexes, extends, rotates and bends, it's sending information to the brain through the central nervous system, or spinal cord, and that's how your brain can understand where you are in time and space. It's this information system that ultimately allows for self-regulation and coordination of all biological and physiological functions of life.

These nerve cells and fibers, as they relate to the brain and how our body self-regulates, affect more tissues than the ones they live in. They have a direct effect on all glands, veins, arteries, muscles, organs, and other tissues of the body. When your spinal joints function properly, your brain will get the essential and unrestricted information it needs to understand the internal physiological world and the external biological environment and be able to maintain each in a cooperative balance.

If you truly want to be optimally well and live a well-adjusted life, it is essential for you to understand the condition called *vertebral subluxation complex* (VSC). A vertebral subluxation is a condition that causes a state of dis-ease, and it's only fully understood, studied, and addressed within the field of chiropractic. There are various people in the scientific and medical realm that are aware of the devastating causes and effects of VSC, but their numbers are few to say the least!

VSC is a global pandemic that affects all human beings from birth to death if it's not detected and corrected with consistency by a Doctor of Chiropractic. With 25 years of active practice and the experience of consulting with several thousand practice members, I can tell you without hesitation or doubt that your health is being affected *at this moment* by one or more vertebral subluxations, and you probably don't even know it. You might not have any signs or symptoms that you'd be able to relate to vertebral subluxations, but if you haven't had regular and consistent full-scope chiropractic care as a regular lifestyle of health care, you're suffering the ill effects of subluxation.

Dr. B.J. Palmer is known as the developer of chiropractic. He took chiropractic from obscurity and defined it as a science, art, and philosophy. In this poem from 1944, he helps to make the reader aware of how a small thing can affect so much:

"A slip on the snowy sidewalk in winter is a small thing. It happens to millions. A fall from a ladder in the summer is a small thing. It also happens to millions. The slip or fall produces a subluxation. The subluxation is a small thing. The subluxation produces pressure on a nerve. That pressure is a small thing. That decreased flowing produces a dis-eased body and brain. That is a big thing to that man (woman/child). Multiply that sick man (woman/child) by a thousand, and you control the physical and mental welfare of a city. Multiply that man (woman/child) by one hundred thirty million, and you forecast and can prophesy the physical and mental status of a nation. So, the slip or fall, the subluxation, pressure, flow of mental images and dis-ease are big enough to control the thoughts and actions of a nation.

Now comes a man (woman). And one man (woman) is a small thing. This man (woman) gives an adjustment. The adjustment is a small thing. The adjustment replaces the subluxation. That is a small thing. The adjusted subluxation releases pressure upon nerves. That is a small thing. The released pressure restores health to a man (woman/child). This is a big thing to that man (woman or child). Multiply that well man (woman/child) by a thousand, and you step up the physical and mental welfare of a city. Multiply that well man (woman or child) by a million, and you increase the efficiency of a state. Multiply that well man (woman/child) by a hundred thirty million, and you have produced a healthy, wealthy, and better race for posterity.

So, the adjustment of the subluxation to release pressure upon nerves, to restore mental impulse flow, to restore health, is big enough to rebuild the thoughts and actions of the world. The idea that knows the cause, that can correct the cause of dis-ease, is one of the biggest ideas known. Without it, nations fall; with it, nations rise. This idea is the biggest I know of."

- B. J. Palmer, 1944

As Doctor of Chiropractic, I've spent over half of my life caring for thousands of people that have suffered from the adverse effects of subluxation, and most didn't even know it until we did a full and comprehensive consultation and specific examination. These people that I've cared for through full-scope chiropractic care would have been much healthier had they been informed and educated to make better choices in lifestyle, and specifically, in spinal and neurological health, much earlier in life. As Dr. B.J. Palmer so eloquently wrote, those practice members would've been better off had we done the adjustment as soon as the subluxation or dis-ease occurred, instead of waiting for it to affect the whole of their life.

Globally, the health care system (more appropriately called a sick care system) is in crisis, and our citizens are sicker than ever before. Real and positive change is possible, but it won't come in the form of more drugs and surgery. In fact, the statistics in the United States alone prove out this point.

In the United States, we are less than 5% of the total global population, yet we consume over 50% of all global prescription drugs annually. The citizens of the United States are prescribed and consume 85% of all globally prescribed opioid pain medications annually. Is it any wonder why our drug epidemic is destroying so many families? We are failing badly by World Health Organization standards for health quality and longevity. These are the statistics that drive me every day, and the reason why I've given 2-1/2 decades of my life to the education, empowerment, and care of my family, my practice members and my communities!

In the next chapter, I'll share the science that supports the subluxation model, and help you understand how VSC is a primary cause of dis-ease, and why it's important to get regular spinal check-ups and chiropractic adjustments, from birth to the last day of life.

I take my role as a doctor very seriously, especially the role I play as an educator! I have deep passion, and I've made a primary commitment to all the communities I practice in, to share this knowledge. I spend much of my time speaking to my colleagues about the responsibility we have to educate our communities more openly, honestly, and with more conviction than ever before. Some of my key commitments and contributions to public education and health safety have been in the co-development of the only spinal hygiene curriculum ever developed to educate children on the importance of spinal health concepts, as well as working with businesses and organizations through the development and implementation of wellness lectures and programs.

Beyond my commitment to community leadership, I've provided safe, specific, scientific, and effective chiropractic care and support to many thousands of individuals and families, to improve their lives. I know without a doubt that this information and the resources I provide to my practice members and community is pivotal to full health expression, and that's why I've chosen to put it up front as one of the first chapters in this book.

Chapter 3

The Spine, The Nervous System, and You

In this chapter, I'll provide a more comprehensive explanation of the cause and effect of VSC. This term describes a condition that is more common, more certain to affect you, and more detrimental to your life than that of heart disease, cavities, high blood pressure, and every other condition you have an understanding of.

VSC is so detrimental, so impactful, and so misunderstood. It is unknown to all health professionals (except Doctors of Chiropractic), and almost always misdiagnosed. You might ask yourself, "How could there be a condition that I've never heard of, or never been told about, that could impact my life so dramatically?" Good question!

VSC affects every aspect of your life and manifests itself in many different ways. For most health professionals, it's a complete unknown, as it is not taught or talked about in standard medical or allied health curriculums.

VSC represents a major obstacle to living a well-adjusted and vital life of optimal health expression. I guarantee VSC is a daily issue affecting you unless or until you commit to a lifestyle of full-scope chiropractic care, to regain and maintain spinal integrity, nervous system adaptability, and physiological homeostasis. Unless and until that time, you will suffer from the escalating effects of VSC and never know it. Don't get me wrong, you will eventually feel the effects of

VSC, but you may never know what the true *cause* of your symptoms are, because it will be called something else, like arthritis, nerve damage, muscle spasm, tendonitis, disc degeneration, or the worst of all "normal aging." Ughhhh!

The term VSC is used almost exclusively by the chiropractic profession to define a spinal vertebra that is misaligned from its normal positioning, fixated in a rigid position, or out of normal juxtaposition with the vertebrae opposing it. This imbalance in structural function in turn causes an interference or distortion of normal nervous system function and a diminished state of adaptability, self-regulation, system controls, and health.

If we break the word subluxation down into its component parts we get *sub* (less than), *lux* (light or energy), and *tion* (condition). By definition, a subluxation is *a condition of less energy or less light.* The information and research I share in this chapter will show how VSC causes a disruption in normal messaging, or a distortion of the information going from the brain to the body and from the body to the brain.

The long-term effects of this diminished or disrupted neurological state creates a lack of adaptability to stress, a reduced ability to coordinate vital systems, and an inability of the body to self-regulate to maintain health. The brain not only controls the internal environment of the body and its systems (including posture, coordination, heart rate, temperature, respiration, digestion, immune function, adaptability, and glandular balance), it's also ultimately responsible for adapting and responding to stressors in our external environment. The central and peripheral nervous systems need to have constant communication to and from brain and the body, and internal and external environments, to create optimal coordination of our complex physiology.

To illustrate how amazing and incredibly adaptable the nervous system is, I'll share a story about life that will no doubt be a familiar one. The difference between living life and becoming aware of its magnitude is awe-inspiring. If you've driven within the last 4-8 hours, it probably seemed like a perfectly mundane experience, not unlike most things you have done thousands of time. But when we break down what was really happening during that drive, you can witness the wonder of YOU! The complexity of what happens during that most mundane and inconsequential last drive will boggle your mind once you drink in the magnitude of coordination it took for you to complete it successfully!

In the course of a normal drive, you're coordinating a multitude of different functions with precision and coordination, with little to no real conscious awareness. You signal left or right in advance at the proper distance of your turn. Your ability to set up the turn in advance with the coordination of signaling allows you to perform a precision left or right turn with accuracy, repeatedly, safely and securely.

You need to brake, accelerate, or coast effectively by monitoring the right amount of pressure on the brake and gas peddles, according to the demands of ever varying traffic patterns and road conditions. You probably turned the radio on and tuned it to your favorite station, listened to a song that reminded you of a very specific time, place, or person, and you felt the emotion that was relevant to that memory.

In normal driving conditions, you have to monitor traffic in 3 different mirrors, change lanes safely and efficiently, adjust the heat or air conditioning, and adjust many other aspects of your environment to suit your comfort. If you had a passenger, you engaged in conversation by interpreting the speed, tone and tempo of their words to determine their intention, understand their perspective, and think through a response that allows you to share your perspective.

As you perform these habitual patterns of action and reactions, your body is regulating your blood pressure, respiration, and digestion, breaking down millions of cells, building up millions of cells, filtering toxins from your blood, and thousands of multifaceted and miraculous physical, mental, and physiological actions.

That's not all folks! You decide what you need to pick up so you can prepare dinner, you make plans to pick up or drop off the kids, and you may remember a task you forgot to do earlier, so you immediately change course to get it done on the way. You also probably adjust your glasses, adjust your seat, drink coffee, and might even be finishing your breakfast! Wow, amazing right? In this illustration it becomes obvious that even in the most "mundane" moments of life you are glorious in your abilities and you don't even realize it!

Because you have a nervous system, you're literally able to complete thousands of different physical, mental, and physiological functions with little to no conscious thought or effort, every moment of every day of your life. As your brain was processing all that information and coordinating your physiological actions and reactions, your body was also adapting to physical, chemical, and mental/emotional stress. Awe inspiring, isn't it?

You don't have to think about these normal functions much because your nervous system is such a miraculous machine. It's so unbelievably responsive and adaptive, it can coordinate a dizzying array of essential functions, activities, actions, reactions, and responses with little to no conscious thought. This capacity is called "unconscious competence," and it's the result of the learned or skilled activities that develop through the repetition and training of your somatic and autonomic nervous systems.

Because you have a nervous system that learns complex patterns of coordination over time and with repetition, your body is able to control and coordinate all the physical and physiological functions necessary for you to navigate life.

Even though the driving illustration is easy to understand, and it highlights the primacy of the nervous system, it doesn't mean that while you successfully accomplished your drive you were expressing optimal function, adaptability, and a complete expression of health. In reality, it's fully possible to experience life with a perceived state of optimal function while at the same time having a state of compensation or dis-ease. When one lives with VSC, the subjective clues (symptoms) may not become obvious until there have been decades of premature aging, imbalances in coordination, a sluggish digestive system, glandular incompetence, a lack of spinal integrity and diminished neurological adaptability.

So far, we've talked mostly about adaptability, and it's time we get to the other side of the coin, which is compensation. If you'll recall, in the last chapter we defined a state of ease as one of balance, adaptability, and homeostasis. The flip side of the coin is the state of dis-ease. Dis-ease is a state of diminished balance, adaptability, and homeostasis. It's important to note that I'm explaining a state of function, not a state of feeling.

You may remember from the last chapter that symptoms are not the first thing to show up when a state of dis-ease goes undetected and uncorrected, but the last. It's normal for most people to feel good for most of their lives while they are functioning poorly. In fact, if you're living in a subluxated state (and I guarantee you are unless you've had regular full-scope chiropractic care from birth), you're in a state of dis-ease right now, which is most likely surprising to hear.

Now that I've explained the effects of subluxation, it's time to fully explain the mechanism of subluxation and how it causes a state of asymptomatic and systematic dis-ease. I'll purposefully leave out a scholarly discussion of the geography of the brain, biochemical reactions, spinal cord tracks, afferent and efferent nerve impulses, antero-grade and retro-grade impulses and the like, as it may be distracting. My hope with this real-world explanation of the mechanisms of subluxation is that you'll understand, without any doubt, the very real and damaging effects of VSC on your human experience.

I truly hope that once you better understand how impactful this condition is you'll see the wisdom in getting checked and corrected through specific, scientific, and safe chiropractic! If so, I'll have accomplished a very critical task as a leader. If you choose not to, I've learned to "be okay" with that. I have a deep sense of responsibility to educate and empower, but I have no control over the decisions others make for their health.

The truth is simple: VSC has a causal relationship to disease through a lack of adaptability to stress, neurological compensation, physiological imbalance, a lack of homeostasis, and diminished health expression. This causal relationship between spinal imbalance, VSC, and a dis-eased state exists whether you understand it or not, whether you believe it or not, and whether you feel it or not.

The causes of subluxation are physical, chemical, and mental/emotional stress that are inherent in every second of every minute of every day of life. Stress is unavoidable, but don't let that depress you. With regular, full-scope chiropractic care we can reduce the likelihood that VSC will lead to full-blown disease! I believe, due to the cause, that the development of VSC is rather unavoidable, but the damage it exacts on your life can be minimized by living a balanced lifestyle. This will be discussed in greater detail in later chapters.

By having regular and consistent spinal and nervous system check-ups in coordination with full-scope chiropractic care, the signs of spinal subluxation can be detected and corrected before they manifest as dis-ease and eventually full-blown disease. When we consider your average daily life from the moment you wake in the morning until the time you go to bed at night, you'll see clearly how stress is ever present and unrelenting.

There are gravitational, chemical, mental/emotional, and physical stresses, as well as past traumas that cause scaring of tissues, loss of normal spinal curves due to poor posture, low levels of movement at work and home, toxins in the air we breathe and the products we use for daily care, and a plethora of other factors that challenge your level of health continuously.

Life in its normal state challenges your body's ability to adapt, it demands constant actions and reactions, and it can and often does interfere with the state of ease, that is, the level of healthy adaptation needed to create and maintain a perfect state of health. I help people understand how life causes subluxation by using an analogy of capacity. As with most analogies, this one should not be taken literally, but when taken figuratively it is spot on.

Imagine the nervous system being a 12 ounce glass. It can only hold 12 ounces of liquid, not 12 ounces plus one drop. In this analogy, let's say the substance the nervous system holds is water, which corresponds to stress. If you were to take that glass and begin putting an ounce of water into it for every life stress, like past trauma, chemical stress (prescription or non-prescription drugs or the use nicotine, caffeine, dehydration), or emotional stress (severe stress in our relationships or our work), these ounces of stress are going to literally reduce the capacity of the nervous system, ultimately diminishing the capacity of the nervous system to manage or hold the amount of life stress pouring in.

When the nervous system is overflowing, it causes VSC, and the chronic nerve interference caused by VSC continues to further diminish the capacity of the nervous system to adapt. I hope this makes sense, because it's a critical concept for your health! When VSC is undetected and uncorrected over days, weeks, months, and years, your ability to manage life is diminished to a point where disease becomes inevitable.

In this analogy, what do you think happens to that extra stress? That's right, it would overflow! Dis-ease is what happens when the overflow occurs. The stress must go somewhere, and the nervous system has to decide where to put it. It doesn't just vanish. Have you ever thought or heard someone say they "carry their stress in their shoulder or their lower back?" That's not the actual truth, but the truth is that is wherever their body absorbs the overflow, that's where there's the most damage, and therefore the least resistance to overflow.

Tissue resistance is a critical factor in adaptation to stress and the maintenance of health as we can see in this example. There are basically 2 different types of tissue in the body, "somatic tissue" and "visceral tissue." The nervous system in its intelligence, whenever possible, will "park" extra stress in somatic tissues (bones, ligaments, tendons, muscle), as a preference to parking it in visceral tissues (liver, spleen, kidney, heart, thyroid, and so on). When the overflow happens, the somatic tissues ultimately lose their strength, flexibility, reliability, and ability to function normally.

When somatic tissue is affected in this way, it becomes a less adequate and reliable tissue as a messenger of mechanical information. This effectively diminishes the information the body can relay to the brain, and the brain can't count on the body to respond adequately. For optimal adaptability and a full health expression the brain and

42

nervous system have to understand the external environment and organize the internal environment of the body.

This restricted nervous system capacity from decreased nerve conduction interferes with the normal messaging from brain to body and body to brain and causes the resulting condition of dis-ease. I'll cover this mechanism later, but for starters, even as over simplified as this explanation is, you start to get a sense of the real-life cause of subluxation.

There are 2 primary mechanisms that cause subluxation to occur. We've addressed the causation from life stress, but there's also a mechanical cause that is related to acute and/or chronic mechanical stress. Often times with the mechanical cause, the symptoms are more immediate, but will go away quickly as the body develops a compensation pattern to deal with the short term acute inflammation or tissue damage.

Most people that suffer with subluxation either symptomatically (with symptoms) or asymptomatically (without symptoms) have both causal factors at play for decades before they ever know it. The most unfortunate folks are the ones that seek standard medical care for acute or chronic symptoms and are given drugs to cover up the symptoms. Unfortunately, our symptom-based health care system prolongs the long-term and damaging cause of the problem by address the short-term symptoms.

If we look at the physiological end state of subluxation, i.e. dis-ease, we can easily show a linear relationship for both development models. When I say linearity, I do so for illustration purposes only, for there is no true linearity in any biological system, especially in the human condition of life. If you understand these flows of "cause," you can see how there's a relationship between structure and physiology that flows both directions.

If we look at subluxation in terms of a mechanical model we get this relationship:

- Structural Instability → Reduced Neurological Input to the Central Nervous System → Altered Physiological Adaptation → Dis-ease

If we look at subluxation from a life stress model we get this relationship:

- Physical, Chemical, Mental/Emotional Stress → Nervous System Overflow → Diminished Somatic Tissue Function → Structural Instability → Reduced Neurological Input to the Central Nervous System → Altered Physiological Adaptation → Dis-ease.

The Neurology of it All

There are multiple types of nerve cells and nerve fibers in the body, the primary of which are motor, sensory, and autonomic. Let's just say that these different fibers or nerve types are the messengers that shape your life experience in every dimension. When they all work together you get ease, but when they don't, you get, you guessed it, dis-ease!

Sensory nerve fibers: The sensory nerve fibers that are responsible for pain sensation are called nociceptors. Nociceptors can be stimulated by chemical, inflammatory, or mechanical irritation, and are responsible for carrying messages from the periphery to the central nervous system and the brain (afferent).

Another critical nerve type in the sensory system is the mechanoreceptor. Mechanoreceptors live in the soft tissues of the body and are primarily responsible for the relay of information about the body's relationship to our external world. They affect the responses needed to manage our internal environment. Sensory nerve cells and fibers are tied directly to the motor and autonomic nerve described below. Don't mistake the word sensory to describe awareness, as most sensory nerve impulses are undetectable, and many sensory impulses never even reach the conscious brain.

Motor nerve fibers: These cause voluntary and involuntary muscles to react to input from the central nervous system going to the periphery (efferent). The motor nerves carry information from the brain to the body and are responsible for muscle coordination, including the tone, quality, and quantity of muscle contraction. Your brain needs the crucial role of the mechanoreceptor to sense position or motion so it can then direct an impulse to the motor nerve fibers that animate the joint and coordinate adaptability.

When a joint moves properly mechanoreceptors fire and tell the brain where you are in relationship to your external environment, and what needs to happen to regulate your internal environment through muscle coordination, balance regulation, structural and postural coordination, ambulation, and overall homeostasis. You get the point, mechanoreceptors are critical to the brain and critical to your health.

Autonomic nerve fibers: The autonomic nervous system controls "automatic" functions (respiration, heart rate, temperature modulation, circulation, and the control of involuntary or smooth muscle in the stomach, esophagus, blood vessels, and so on). Like the other type of nerve fibers discussed above, the autonomic nervous system is sensitive to inputs and outcomes from the external and internal environments.

The autonomic nervous system has 2 distinct parts: the sympathetic (fight or flight) and the parasympathetic (rest and digest). Balanced adaptability to stress and the expression of optimal well-being requires a balance between the sympathetic and the parasympathetic nervous systems. The autonomic nervous system is directly affected by increased nociceptive activity or decreased mechanoreceptor activity that stems from the joint complex.

The autonomic nervous system is directly affected by VSC by the following means: it moves toward a sympathetic (fight or flight) or parasympathetic (rest and digest) condition as a result of the quality and quantity of the information it gets from the nociceptor and mechanoreceptor fibers of the sensory nervous systems.

When the autonomic nervous system has a reduction of mechanoreceptor activity you get a resultant increase in nociceptive activity, as mechanoreceptor activity has a diminishing effect of nociceptor amplitude. This reduction in mechanoreceptor activity occurs when the joint is fixated, as in the case of the VSC.

With VSC, you get reduced mechanoreceptor activation, increased nociceptor activity and sympathetic dominance (fight or flight) in the body physiologically. As a result of the fight or flight condition, the body releases stress hormones called cortisol and adrenalin, which are "no bueno" for optimal long-term health expression.

Cortisol and adrenalin are very potent chemicals that serve an essential role in our survival mechanism of life. They enhance our ability to run, jump, react, and flee from danger. The problem with the chronic and unrelenting release of cortisol and adrenalin, which happens in the disease state of subluxation, is that it hinders our normal physiological patterns of circulation, hormonal balance, muscle coordination, cardiac function, digestion and all other cellular and systems regulation.

Fight or flight is an essential need if you are being chased by a bear, but it's incredibly damaging in ordinary life, living an average lifestyle. If there's a case for the importance for living a lifestyle that includes full-scope chiropractic care, the connection between joint function and autonomic balance is a good one!

If we look at subluxation in terms of a mechanical model we get this relationship:

Structural Instability → Reduced Neurological Input to the Central Nervous System → Altered Physiological Adaptation → Dis-ease.

If we look at subluxation from a life stress model we get this relationship:

Physical, Chemical, Mental/Emotional Stress → Nervous System Overflow → Diminished Somatic Tissue Function → Structural Instability → Reduced Neurological Input to the Central Nervous System → Altered Physiological Adaptation → Dis-ease.

In the mechanical and stress models I highlighted above, you can clearly see that structural instability can begin the cascade of the neurological and physiological dis-ease patterns that cause the subluxation complex.

In review: joint fixation and a lack of motion in a tissue (joint) → diminished mechanoreceptor activation → increase influence of nociceptors on the brain → a state of sympathetic dominance (fight or flight) → vasoconstriction and a stagnation of chemicals locally in the joint → acceleration of nociceptor (pain) signaling → further reduced mechanoreceptor activation → muscle splinting → increased joint fixation and reduction of motion (joint) → the loop continues.

If you think this sounds bad, this fixation degeneration (arthritis) is just what happens in the joint complex and the nervous system locally. The most damaging effect on your long-term health is how this causes overall exhaustion on your body's ability to understand your environment, organize adaptive responses to stress, and organization global responses that are necessary to thrive. If we look at the effects of VSC beyond the local effect, it's not hard to see how it can interfere with the normal function of our critical systems and organs: thyroid gland, pituitary gland, our endocrine system, circulatory system, cardiovascular system, liver, spleen, digestive system, and so on.

The basic truth (I say basic, as it would be far too in depth to discuss it in specific neurological and physiological terms) is this: when you're in fight or flight, your body is in a state of protection, and the body cannot be in a perpetual state of protection and be in a robust state of repair at the same time.

When the body is in a chronic stress pattern due to VSC, it can't heal or repair at the speed that the body breaks down. Living in a chronic state of VSC weakens the immune response, slows the body's repair mechanism, diminishes our adaptive potential, and therefore diminishes our expression of vital health and optimal well-being. To be redundant, that condition is called a state of dis-ease.

Now you understand how subluxation is caused by physical, chemical, mental/emotional stress that is present at a higher quantity or capacity than the body can adapt to. The altered or compensated state of VSC becomes a feedback loop of decreased mechanoreceptor activity, increased nociceptor activity, increased motor tone or splinting of the joint which leads to degenerative arthritis and increased sympathetic dominance. This causes vasoconstriction, glandular disruption, increased cardiovascular stress, and the hits go on.

All major killers like cancer, diabetes, heart disease, degenerative arthritis (yes, degenerative arthritis in its end stage reduces quality and quantity of life), are preventable in most cases, as they are nothing more than dis-ease that went undetected and uncorrected for too long.

In later chapters we'll talk about the importance of lifestyle as an essential tool in the development of an optimally healthy life, but for now, it's important to understand without doubt that active, flexible, and mobile joints are a critical necessity in the maintenance of proper structure, neurology, and physiology.

To live a life well-adjusted, you must have direct and complete neurological messaging from the brain to the body and the body to the brain. This clear information pathway ensures that your nervous system can understand your external environment, regulate your internal environment, manage your actions/reactions/responses, and maintain a state where all the regulatory systems can promote a full expression of adaptability and self-healing.

I think I've made it abundantly clear, but, in case I haven't, I'll make a final statement on the importance of regular, safe, specific, and scientific full-scope chiropractic care: if you're not using regular, full-scope chiropractic care as part of a wellness lifestyle, from birth to your last day on earth, you're living in a state of dis-ease. Put another way, if you have VSC, you have stress that is not being adapted to meet your body's needs, and you're getting sicker every day. That's just the way it is, and it isn't any other way!

If you're subluxated, which is certainly the case, you don't have the vital health I am sure you desire, and that I believe you deserve. With a subluxated spinal system, you're compensating, not adapting. You're getting sicker, not healthier, you're getting weaker, not stronger. If we want to live *A Life Worth Living*, a life that's well-adjusted, we must start with the master systems of the body, the spinal and nervous systems.

By reading this far, you've already learned more about the relationship between the spine and your health than 90% of the population. It's distressing to me that most people still believe chiropractic to be only good for neck or back pain, and quite frankly it's about this concern that I write and share my knowledge so often and openly with the public. There are few things further from the truth than the idea that chiropractic is merely a modality to be used in the "treatment" of neck or back pain. It's true that most anyone that experiences back or neck pain can get relief using chiropractic care, but that is the least benefit they get.

Millions of adults and children achieve amazing whole health benefits annually in the U.S and abroad every day from chiropractic. The most amazing effects of living a full-scope chiropractic lifestyle come from the body's ability to resolve health conditions that are seemingly unrelated to the spine. Chiropractic doesn't treat any condition other than VSC, but the body has an extraordinary ability to heal and self-regulate when VSC is reduced, and the body regains a state of optimal adaptability or ease. For this reason, everyone deserves the chance to have their spine and nervous system checked and cared for by a chiropractor!

Using medicine to treat symptoms or using pain-based (limited-scope) chiropractic care for the sole purpose of treating the symptoms of neck or back pain would be like waking up at 2am to a fire alarm and merely removing the batteries so you can go back to bed without being bothered to find out why it was going off in the first place.

I hesitate to use an example that is as specific as the following study results, but I want to share the findings so you can better understand how other critical systems are effected by VSC.

"Chiropractic spinal adjustments improve digestive function by reducing interference in the central nervous system and the related function of the systems it controls and regulates. The 2009 study published in the European Journal of Gastroenterology and Hepatology (below) found that the relationship between vertebral subluxation complex and digestive system disorders is directly related. This study is simple and straight-forward involving the significance of chiropractic spinal adjustments and digestive health. Chiropractors performed spinal adjustments on 83 patients over a 2-year period. The 83 patients that were evaluated had symptoms of digestive pain in the chest and epigastric area for more than 2 years."

Here are the results:

"The patients were treated conservatively with chiropractic adjustments and soft tissue techniques. 71% of the patients reported an improvement in the average severity of their symptoms. No patients reported any worsening of their symptoms and 45% reported they reduced their use of dyspepsia drugs. This study has indicated that chiropractic adjustments can have a significant positive effect on digestive pain."

The Power of Paradigm

Paradigm: a framework containing the basic assumptions, ways of thinking, and methodology that are commonly accepted by members of a scientific community.

Source: Dictionary.com

If you want to experience true healing in any "care" program, it must start with a paradigm that is based on an initial premise that leads to the thoughts and actions that will lead to the outcome you desire. The biggest problem we face in our current sick care system is the paradigm and vision. Our sick care system is symptom based. It's defined, designed, and directed to "treat" the subjective experience of the patient, not to detect and correct the objective findings of disease. Therefore, the eventual outcome is sickness without symptoms, and not a return to health. If the focus of care is the treatment of disease, you will not end with more health, you will end with less disease.

Consider this: health and sickness are like light and dark respectively. The condition of health (light) is created by the *presence of energy* and the condition of sickness (dark) is created by the *absence of energy*. You cannot create health by reducing sickness, you can only create health by adding energy to the system. Conversely, the only way to create sickness is by taking energy away from the system.

In practical terms, the only way to get rid of sickness is to improve health, not treat the sickness. A physician friend of mine summed it up perfectly when he told me that the practice of medicine is great at taking the individual from a state of -10 to 0 on the sickness scale but fails miserably at taking an individual form 0 to + 10 on a health scale.

To highlight the difference between healthcare (proactive) and sick care (reactive), I'd like to share this poem authored by Joseph Malins in 1895. After reading it you may ask yourself the question I ask myself daily: why do we (123 years after the authorship of this poem) continue to focus on the treatment of disease instead of on the promotion of health?

An Ambulance Down in The Valley

'Twas a dangerous cliff, as they freely confessed,
Though to walk near its crest was so pleasant;
But over its terrible edge there had slipped
A duke and full many a peasant.
So the people said something would have to be done,
But their projects did not at all tally;
Some said, "Put a fence 'round the edge of the cliff,"
Some, "An ambulance down in the valley."

But the cry for the ambulance carried the day,
For it spread through the neighboring city;
A fence may be useful or not, it is true,
But each heart became full of pity.
For those who slipped over the dangerous cliff;
And the dwellers in highway and alley,
Gave pounds and gave pence, not to put up a fence,
But an ambulance down in the valley.

"For the cliff is all right, if you're careful," they said,
"And, if folks even slip and are dropping,
It isn't the slipping that hurts them so much
As the shock down below when they're stopping."
So day after day, as these mishaps occurred,
Quick forth would those rescuers sally,
To pick up the victims who fell off the cliff,
With their ambulance down in the valley.

Then an old sage remarked: "It's a marvel to me
That people give far more attention
To repairing results than to stopping the cause,
When they'd much better aim at prevention.
Let us stop at its source all this mischief," cried he,
"Come, neighbors and friends, let us rally;
If the cliff we will fence, we might almost dispense
With the ambulance down in the valley."

"Oh he's a fanatic," the others rejoined,
"Dispense with the ambulance? Never!
He'd dispense with all charities, too, if he could;
No! No! We'll support them forever.
Aren't we picking up folks just as fast as they fall?
And shall this man dictate to us? Shall he?
Why should people of sense stop to put up a fence,
While the ambulance works in the valley?"

But the sensible few, who are practical too,
Will not bear with such nonsense much longer;
They believe that prevention is better than cure,
And their party will soon be the stronger.
Encourage them then, with your purse, voice, and pen,
And while other philanthropists dally,
They will scorn all pretense, and put up a stout fence
On the cliff that hangs over the valley.

Better guide well the young than
      reclaim them when old,
For the voice of true wisdom is calling.
"To rescue the fallen is good, but 'tis best
To prevent other people from falling."
Better close up the source of temptation and crime
Than deliver from dungeon or galley;
Better put a strong fence 'round the top of the cliff
Than an ambulance down in the valley.

What is full-scope chiropractic care? Full-scope chiropractic care starts with a willingness to seek true healthcare and a desire to venture outside the typical medical model of symptom-focused relief care. A complete care cycle in a full-scope chiropractic model has a beginning, a middle, but no end. You'll see that a proper full-scope chiropractic program goes far beyond a symptom review and prescription, as happens in most medical environments.

It includes:

- A complete consultation including history, current health status, future health goals, and expectations for outcomes.

- A complete examination including postural assessment, spinal palpation, range of motion testing, neurological evaluation, spinal integrity testing, and x-ray.

- A report of findings which is critical to tie together the consultation, the examination, and to plan the proper care plan to result in the expected health outcomes as defined in the consultation.

Track 1: Physical and Physiological Well-Being

Acute Phase

The acute phase of care is designed to be a short-term initial (first phase) approach to full-scope chiropractic care, with the goal of disrupting pain patterns, reducing inflammation, promoting healthy movement patterns, reducing neurological interference, and beginning the healing process by increasing brain body communication patterns. This phase of care is defined by high frequency of care for a short duration. Acute care typically lasts 4-12 weeks depending on the overall quality of spinal tissue and structure, the quantity of compensation structurally and neurologically, and the ability of the individual to heal.

Acute care is an essential beginning to full-scope chiropractic care, but as a standalone care plan its long-term value to overall health creation is limited and not long standing. This is where standard medical approaches end and why they fail to create any long-term health changes. When the primary focus is on the symptoms of dis-ease, the cause of disease is never addressed, and the creation of health never occurs.

Rehabilitative Phase

The rehabilitative phase of care is designed to further promote full body healing by reinforcing proper spinal integrity and neurological balance. In the rehabilitative phase of care, symptoms are usually gone, the body is adapting to stress better, the tissues are under repair, and the balance and homeostasis of optimal wellness is being established.

Rehabilitative care typically lasts longer than the acute phase, with a reduced frequency of care. The rehabilitative phase of care is an extension of the early work of acute care. It takes the healing factor to a new level as it allows for the time necessary for the body to unwind compensation patterns and regain and maintain optimal adaptation patterns to stress.

Wellness Phase

The wellness phase of care should be thought of as a lifestyle approach to regaining and maintaining optimal spinal, neurological, and physiological health and well-being. In the wellness phase, the structure and neurology have been optimized, and the brain and body are communicating with great clarity and coordination. Optimized does not necessarily mean perfect, as the condition of the tissue determines the degree of healing that is possible for each individual. In the 33 principles of chiropractic we understand matter can be a limiting factor in healing.

The frequency of care is reduced but consistent. The wellness phase of full-scope chiropractic care is designed to maintain health (ease) instead of treating a condition (dis-ease). In the wellness phase of care, the focus will include other factors of lifestyle that influence adaptability and overall health expression. Wellness-focused chiropractic care has no defined end, but the focus will be different than it was in the acute and rehabilitative care phases. If one fails to regain optimal health and maintain it with regular and consistent wellness care, dis-ease and the potential for disease patterns is inevitable.

To draw a close to this chapter, I would like to share a piece written by Dr. Jeremy Book, one of the managing partners of the Chiropractic Vitality Centers of Maine and the leader of our Innate Chiropractic team in Portland Maine. In defining what chiropractic is, he likes to explain one of the more powerful truths in healthcare, the concept of "Above, Down, Inside, Out" (ADIO).

"A.D.I.O. is an acronym coined by Dr. B.J. Palmer, the developer of the chiropractic profession. Dr. Palmer not only developed the practice of chiropractic, he defined the philosophy that set the paradigm it is practiced under. The "backbone" of chiropractic philosophy is the concept of "innate intelligence." Innate intelligence is the intelligence "within" that controls every single action and reaction that occurs within our bodies. It all starts with conception. When a sperm cell and egg cell come together how do they know to form a human? Innate intelligence. This intelligence continues to live within us and allows our body to perform tasks without us having to think about them. For example, the beating of your heart, the regulation of breathing, or the healing of a cut on your hand are all examples of your innate intelligence at work.

As a chiropractor, I understand that innate intelligence is smarter than any doctor ever could be. Your body always knows what is best for it when innate intelligence is able to flow from body to brain and brain to body without interference. This innate intelligence is expressed in our bodies via the nervous system.

The role of chiropractic care is to balance the nervous system, freeing the spine and nerves from interference, allowing innate intelligence to flow optimally. The nervous system is comprised of your spine, spinal cord, and an extensive network of peripheral nerves that control every single organ, tissue, and cell. The intelligence comes from your brain, travels down your spinal cord, and then out to each part of your body.

Most people underestimate the ability of their body to heal, however, true healing ONLY comes from within. No magic potion, powder, or drug can ever replace innate intelligence and its ability to heal the body. We know that true health comes from Above, Down, Inside, Out. Chiropractors have recognized this fact for 123 years."

- Contributed by Dr. Jeremy Book

As a Chiropractor with 25 years' experience, I deeply desire to be a good leader for my community, a worthy coach for those that want more health than sickness, and a great doctor and strong advocate for my practice members. (I don't use the term patient as it literally means "one who suffers.") It's my goal with the writing of this book that you'll get a better sense of my "priorities" as they relate to the care I provide and the focus I give to structure and neurology.

As a result of the information in this book, I hope we're both fortunate enough to work together as doctor and practice member. If we do, there will be a major focus on spinal and neurological health. If we don't accomplish that, then we fail to set the foundation for the conscious, purposeful, value-based, goal-centered, and action-oriented life you deserve, a life that I call "My Life Well-Adjusted."

Chapter 4

Health and Sickness are 2 Sides

of the Same Coin

The difference between health and sickness is so important to understand that I'll spend this chapter helping you make critical distinctions that can determine the outcomes of your health for life. Let's start by digging a little deeper into the concept of health being the equivalent of light, and sickness being that of darkness. This analogy can be a tricky one, so bear with me as I use a slightly different style of phrasing to establish a clear point regarding the difference between health/ease (presence of light and energy) and sickness/dis-ease (the absence of light and energy).

To understand light and energy exchanges in a biological world is fundamental to defining the optimal or sub-optimal states of tissue health, structural integrity, physiological balance and overall expression of health in both a microscopic (cellular) and macroscopic (whole system) framework.

You'll remember in this analogy, when using light as a synonym for health/ease and darkness as a synonym for sickness/dis-ease, health is the presence of light and disease if the absence of light. You could also use the word energy instead of light and understand it this way. Health is the presence of energy and disease is the absence of energy.

If you have disease in your life in any dimension it is because there is a lack of light/energy as it is the condition of absence of energy. Health/ease is the presence of light/energy and sickness/dis-ease is the absence of light/energy. Disease does not exist in the presence of total light or the full expression of energy in a biological system and the same can be said for health. Health cannot exist in a biological system that has a lack of light or energy.

Our sick care system fails for a very specific reason: the focus is on removing sickness instead of creating health. To continue this train of logic, our sick care model is a system that tries to create health/light by taking away sickness/dark and there is no way to create health/light by removing sickness/dark!

To develop health, you must focus on health creation and not disease elimination. This makes sense, doesn't it? Phew! I will state it again as I cannot state it with enough emphasis: our sick care system is focused on removing sickness, with little to no emphasis on adding or creating health, and that is precisely why we are seeing greater failures in our health statistics with each generation.

Your state of health is a reflection of your state of energy in quality, quantity, tone, and flow. Energy, as it relates to your overall capacity to adapt to stress and function at the highest level, is an expression of intelligence. True health/ease in its most robust form is created through full and uninterrupted adaptation to physical, chemical, and mental/emotional stress.

Health/ease then is an outcome, not a state, as is true for sickness/dis-ease. Health is the outcome of optimal performance, robust adaptability, and proper self-regulation of all systems (glandular, hormonal, structural, neurological, visceral, and somatic). Health, as you'll recall from the last chapter, is the result of the full expression of the inner intelligence or "innate intelligence" of the body. Health/ease is the side of the lifestyle coin which I believe that we all desire and deserve, but it does not happen by chance, it happens on purpose.

Sickness/dis-ease is the opposite side of the lifestyle outcomes coin, and it's a condition created by the absence of something, not the presence of something. The absence of what? If you said light, energy or intelligence, you are spot on, A+!! Sickness/dis-ease is the absence of energy. It's the absence of self-regulation, spinal integrity, neurological adaptability, and the full and unrestricted flow of intelligence from the body to the brain and the brain to the body. Health and sickness, then, are both outcomes, but they're antithetical, or complete opposite sides of the lifestyle outcomes coin.

You'll learn more about this topic in later chapters, but I'll touch on it briefly now. Until recently, it was believed that our genes were responsible for and/or "caused" most diseases. What we know now is much more enlightened: we now know that 85% of disease patterns are related to lifestyle, not genetics, which to me is empowering!

The health side of the lifestyle coin is an outcome created by consistent inputs of 3 powerful lifestyle divisions: eating well, moving well, and thinking well. Health is the presence of consistent and persistent behavior that reinforces the condition that allows for the expression of intelligence and adaptability, where homeostasis and balance are expressed in optimal function. Good inputs create good outcomes, bad inputs create bad outcomes.

Get ready, I am going to say it again: "Health is the accumulation of good, robust inputs into a living system which allows the presence of healthy, strong, vibrant, vital adaptations to physical, chemical, mental/emotional stress." I know that I've said that often and you can be certain I will say it again. Wait until we meet, it is my "clarion call!" I believe this understanding is so important a concept to your future health that it bears repeating as often as necessary or until it becomes your paradigm of health.

Health in the "move well" dimension of life is the outcome of consistent patterns of movement that challenge the "soft" and "hard" tissues of the body, and require the movement of fluid, energy, and intelligence. When we "move well," it challenges the nervous system to learn patterns of activity that lend to intelligent growth and balance.

Health in the "eat well" dimension of life is the outcome of eating, digestion, and assimilation of proper foods and nutrients on a consistent basis. There are very few areas of health that seem to cause more confusion than nutrition, especially in the realm of weight management and control. In the "My Life Well-Adjusted" program, we deal with this with clear and disciplined approaches to find and fit our members with a program of life-style nutrition, and if necessary, weight loss using the Chirothin doctor-supervised weight loss program.

Lastly, health in the "think well" dimension of life is the outcome of consistent and persistent healthy, optimistic, hopeful, and creative thought patterns that challenge the emotional and intellectual brain and initiate the release of hormones that lead to healthy immune responses and proper glandular activity.

In the end, health/ease or sickness/dis-ease are 2 sides of the same coin. The side that expresses itself in our lives is dependent upon lifestyle inputs, as the inputs will determine the outcomes. A lifestyle that is vital, energetic and adaptive is the key to the expression of intelligence and the expression of intelligence is the cornerstone of health, and ultimately what is required to live a life well-adjusted.

It may seem too simple to be true, but it's not. The simple truth is that health is the presence of great inputs and great outcomes, and sickness is the absence of great inputs and great outcomes. I'd be elated from this day forward if you understand with absolute certainty that your health is in your hands! Your future state of health is not a fateful "luck of the draw" that determines whether you are healthy or sick. It's more a determined state of outcomes that you get to control at least 85% of the time! When we look at human existence in a biological sense, we're looking at pure potential that starts at birth. It's through lifestyle that we create sickness/dis-ease, and it's through lifestyle that we can create health/ease.

We have a choice every day of whether we're going to think empowering, strong vital thoughts or downtrodden, disappointed negative thoughts. We have a choice of whether to move our bodies in ways that are consistent with the outcomes of structural and neurological coordination daily. There are hundreds of opportunities every day for us to make choices for better or worse; choose wisely! The "My Life Well-Adjusted" program was created and is delivered to help you build a highly conscious, well-defined, and purposefully designed life of outcomes that you desire and deserve! If you want to be healthier than you are right now, YOU CAN BE!

Better health is yours to create. When I say create, I mean it's a future-paced concept that is created by current thoughts, actions, and outcomes. The health you deserve and desire doesn't require that you start with the ideal weight or the ideal size. It doesn't matter if you've had challenges in the past - who hasn't?

We can all accomplish a better state of health regardless of the obstacles in our past or the hurdles we must overcome. What it really takes to build better health outcomes is a deep commitment to start AND a willingness to keep going. It is literally shocking to my practice members when they take the "My Life Well-Adjusted" journey and find themselves breaking through the habits and experiences from their past, and beginning to build a new future of clarity and purposeful living.

"My Life Well-Adjusted," *A Life Worth Living* is a creative process of writing the story of your future with clarity, passion, pure consciousness, and absolute purpose. It is not easy, but oh is it worth it! As Napoleon Hill stated, "Whatever the mind of man can conceive and believe, it can achieve!" Do you believe you can build the life that most only dream of? I do, and I want to help you live the life that's most fulfilling and meaningful to you.

Chapter 5

Eat Well, Move Well, Think Well for Life

There are many different terms to describe health being bantered around in society and in the "health care" industry these days. It's not just from providers, but it's also from nutrition firms, super markets, and pharmaceutical companies. Some of the more common terms to describe a state of health are well, optimal, whole, vital, etc. You've heard them all, but they're never really qualified. As a non-qualified or non-quantified entity, they're usually nothing more than sales slogans.

To make a term more than a slogan, to make it real and tangible, it must be meaningful, specific, and attainable. In this chapter, I'll describe the 3 real life dimensions that are necessary to create overall health and well-being. These 3 dimensions have the power to help you create meaningful, specific, and attainable health. If these aren't well thought about or designed, the result can be the development of sickness, disease, and ultimately, early death.

Eat well

It's pretty obvious what that means, right? Maybe not when there are a million different theories, opinions, and methods of "eating well." With all the options available and all the opinions that are thrown around, how do we wade through the confusion to figure out what it means to eat well? It's simple if we break it down to the basic biological needs for the building blocks of life.

The basic building blocks are necessary for the creation and maintenance of the quantity and quality of our cells, systems, immune function, brain health, bone structure, skin health, and strength and coordination in general. The basic needs of the body that we get from diet are essential amino acids, vitamins, minerals, proteins, fats, and carbohydrates.

Some of the phrases that are thrown around about nutrition are helpful, but they don't define what a healthy diet is. For instance, have you ever heard the saying, "eat foods that are more alive than dead if you want to be more alive than dead"? Or, "if it doesn't rot, don't eat it", meaning if it has a long "shelf life" then it's not really food, and it won't contribute in a meaningful way to your health. Or worse, it will create toxicity in the body.

There are as many different diets as there are concepts about nutrition. There's the Mediterranean diet, the whole food diet, the vegan diet, the vegetarian diet, the ketogenic diet, the South Beach diet, and hundreds more! Whatever your desired style of eating is or what your primary philosophy is, there is a diet to fit you.

What we know about the Eat Well concept is that everybody's needs are a little different, based on their lifestyle, how active or inactive they are, how healthy their gut is (often times relating to antibiotic use or overall nutritional content), how hydrated or dehydrated they are, and whether they weight train or focus more on cardiovascular exercise. Or it may depend on other issues such as allergies, preferences, or simply taste.

To say the least, the Eat Well concept can be very confusing and confounding. Some of the suggestions I make are quite general and simple but can make a profound difference if followed:

- Eat foods that are locally harvested, and when possible, organic.

- Eat foods that will rot if they're not consumed in a certain amount of time. That ensures a more living, vital food source.

- If it comes in a box, bag, or can, find a natural source that will be less toxic. (When you have toxicity in the body, the body will expand the fat cells for better storage of toxins).

- Eat around the perimeter. The perimeter of the supermarket traditionally contains the freshest options available. Produce and meats are typically kept cool and peripherally in the market.

- Choose frozen over canned. If you don't have time or for whatever reason can't prepare vegetables and need a quick solution, frozen vegetables are almost categorically superior to canned vegetables. Canned vegetables are generally loaded with salt and tend to have been sitting around longer. Fruits and vegetables are flash frozen and closer to the original product in nutritional content.

- Shop on a full stomach. When we shop hungry we tend to make more impulse buys and poorer choices than if we're satiated. Hint: eat a healthy lunch, breakfast, or snack before you go shopping for your groceries.

Eating well can be difficult due to life circumstances, but it doesn't have to be confusing! Eating a high percentage of complete foods that are digestible is essential so your body can maintain healthy cellular and neurological function, healthy coordination of systems, consistent development of muscular tissue, bony structure, cartilage production, and adaptability to stress.

Lastly, it's important to think about food from a brain perspective. Real whole foods cross the blood-brain barrier and create nutrition for the axons and nerve endings in the brain. Healthy food leads to overall higher levels of adaptability to physical, chemical, and mental/emotional stress.

Move Well

The relationship between movement and health is under-thought, under-spoken and under-taught in our society. Usually we think of movement in the form of stretching, walking, jogging, lifting weights, or participating in sports. What we're generally not fully aware of is the deep and powerful effect of movement as it relates to our expression of health, in both quality and quantity.

Probably the number one question that I get from practice members who come into my chiropractic office with a specific complaint of joint pain is this one: "Is there a set of stretches that I can do to solve this problem?"

The answer is, "No!" There isn't a set of stretches that solves any problems. Stretches can temporarily "short circuit" pain as perceived by the brain, temporarily reduce muscle tension, and facilitate short-term reduction in inflammation, but stretching is an incomplete process, as it doesn't get to the deepest levels of neurological messaging.

The big problems with the concept of stretching is that it's taught to be done reactively and that it's somehow corrective. As a reactive measure, it can aid in recovery locally and systemically, but as a standalone activity, it's focused on a short-term outcome, which leads to short term results.

Based on our history with stretching, it's most often done only when we have a tight muscle or a stiff joint. In the end, if you only do stretches when you have a tight muscle or a stiff joint, you'll end up with more tight muscles and stiff joints. It sounds like a paradox, but it's the truth.

The symptoms of a tight muscle or a stiff joint tells us something is out of balance and that the body is in a state of compensation. If we look beyond the symptom and focus on a complete and proactive assessment of the cause, we can correct the real issue, and not just react to or reduce the symptoms.

Stretching is appropriate and powerful if done proactively from the beginning of life and in coordination with a balanced lifestyle. In fact, movement in the form of stretching can be a vital component to maintaining a healthy relationship between joint function and physiological balance, but stretching alone will not correct or prevent vertebral subluxation complex.

Remember the vertebral subluxation complex from Chapter 1? In case you've forgotten, VSC is a complex structural, neurological, and physiological condition that is most often present without any awareness or early symptoms. VSC affects the adaptability mechanisms of the joint locally and the whole body globally. A lack of normal multidirectional movement (flexion, extension, rotation, and lateral bending), whether it's in a specific joint or the whole body, reduces your life expression. Movement is absolutely key to overall health!

Let's go back and recall the nerve fibers called mechanoreceptors and how key nerve fibers affect other critical adaptive needs. A mechanoreceptor is a type of nerve fiber that feeds the brain with information about time and space. For there to be proper body-brain and brain-body communication, your brain needs to know where you are in time and space.

There are other sensory inputs to the brain that provide awareness and adaptability, like the eyes, ears, and sense of touch, but the mechanoreceptors that live in the joint complex are absolutely essential for creating adaptability in the body.

If optimal adaptation to stress and vital well-being is not enough to emphasize the need for a balanced spine, here are 20 good reasons to get moving:

1. It's good for your heart
2. Exercise promotes weight loss
3. Exercise prevents osteoporosis
4. Exercise lowers high blood pressure
5. Exercise is an excellent de-stressor
6. Exercise prevents colds
7. Exercise reduces the severity of asthma
8. Exercise reduces diabetic complications
9. Exercise promotes a healthy pregnancy
10. Exercise plays a role in preventing cancer
11. Exercise has anti-aging effects
12. Exercise promotes brain health
13. Exercise is great for your sex life
14. Exercise improves sleeping patterns

15. Exercise combats impotence

16. Exercise helps prevent stroke

17. Exercise is good for mind and soul

18. Exercise improves oxygen and nutrient supply to all cells in your body

19. Exercise allows you to improve muscle strength, joint structure and joint function

20. Exercise helps to manage arthritis

Source: www.health24.com

One last key, positive effect of movement is how you look and feel about yourself. If you've noticed your clothes may not fit like they used to, or you have a closet full of the clothes you will be wearing when you lose a couple of pounds, you're not alone. More and more we hear the bad news regarding Americans and obesity, but there is good news too! The good news is that it takes very little time or effort to change your current health status with regard to your weight and your waistline.

Gaining weight and the associated effect on your health is a process that occurs over time and is usually the result of a combination of factors. The most common factors are the perceived lack of time, or a lack of knowledge about how to create a workout routine or nutrition plan that will help you realize the results you want. This double whammy leads to procrastination and a sense of helplessness or defeat.

The second most common reason is the lack of clearly defined goals, and an action plan that includes a realistic timeline for you to achieve your health or fitness goals. These 2 factors often result in choosing a quick fix fad diet, or an overly aggressive exercise program that is too demanding, and not the right fit for the individual. Having clearly defined goals in place for a program of exercise that fits your busy life will lead to a transformation of your health and lead to a more balanced lifestyle.

The most important aspect of getting fit is coming to terms with what is keeping you from getting started. If it's time, it only takes minutes per day for you to start increasing your level of activity. For instance, taking 1,000 extra steps per day will add up to 7000 per week, 28,000 per month and 336,000 per year. For the average person, that would equal 666 miles of walking per year. Imagine the cardiovascular, bone density, and immune benefits. In other words, *you are literally minutes away from the new you!*

If it's confusion on whether to focus on cardiovascular exercise or weight training, ask a fitness expert, or search an online source. At Bangor Family Chiropractic, I always recommend a combination of the 2 for overall health and fitness as part of the "My Life Well-Adjusted" program. If you need help in defining what your current health status is and creating achievable goals, I recommend seeking the help of a full-scope chiropractor who can help you design your health outcomes and guide you to great resources in your community.

Regardless of where you live, there are many different facilities that specialize in health and fitness training, as well as one-on-one coaching. You can join a standalone gym, use the YMCA, seek one-on-one personal training, find a women's fitness studio, do Pilates, yoga, martial arts, or just go for a stroll along the river or a nearby beach.

A proper exercise and fitness program should always start with a comprehensive full-scope chiropractic evaluation to find out if your nerves, muscles, and joints are balanced and functioning properly. For safety and the best results possible, your nervous system and skeletal system need to be balanced and adaptable, otherwise you could develop acute or chronic injuries that spoil your best laid plans.

Please make sure that you and everyone you care about gets checked and adjusted for VSC by a chiropractor with consistency and regularity from birth to their final days. Regular, consistent full-scope chiropractic checkups and adjustments will ensure proper mechanoreceptor activation, proper feeding of the brain, and proper adaptability of the body for the fullest expression of health achievable.

Think Well

The first chapter of the book "Think and Grow Rich" by Napoleon Hill is titled "Thoughts are Things." This chapter is a powerful piece of reading if you want to develop a keen sense of the power of thought! I'll summarize by stating the basic premise: *The outcomes of your life are based on your thoughts.*

Your thoughts are real. They drive your emotions, your physiology, your creativity, and ultimately, they are the foundation for your actions and outcomes in life. Your emotions are often attached to your thoughts, and believe it or not, emotions play a large role in your health.

There have been many studies over the years that show the effect of emotional health and the power of thought on our bodies. It has been universally found that emotions, good and bad, have an impact on our overall state of health. Emotional stress is a natural aspect of life that cannot be avoided, either situationally or in times of trauma, but it can be adapted to healthier outcomes by renegotiating our perspectives on events.

Our emotional thought tendencies impact our immune function, brain chemistry, blood sugar levels, hormone balance and so much more. Have you ever heard the phrase, "she died of a broken heart?" Studies show there is merit to that statement. After losing a loved one, your chances of having a heart attack increase by 21 times. That sounds unbelievable, right?

Our thoughts, and as a result, our emotional state is so connected to our physiology, some scientists suggest using probiotics as a potential alternative to antidepressant medications due to the connection between mood and gut health.

In a study done by Dr. Sheldon Cohen, PhD, he assessed 193 subjects to determine their level of positive emotions (including happiness, calmness, and liveliness). In the study, when he exposed test subjects to a virus, he found that people who scored low on positive emotions were 3 times as likely to succumb to the bug. This is a great study showing that we do have some control over our health, and it can be, in part, as easy as having a positive outlook!

How can you increase the positivity in your life? Here are 5 categories that can go a long way to improving the positivity in your life:

1. Exercise: Exercise is a natural way to release endorphins into your brain. Endorphins have a tranquilizing effect on our physiology through the changes they create in brain chemistry, and how the brain dictates function globally in the body.

2. Restorative sleep: Sleep is so important, you could do everything in life necessary to be healthy, but if you aren't sleeping well your mental health will suffer. Your body needs

good, deep sleep every night to heal and rejuvenate from your day's activities.

3. Meditation: Meditation is a good way to pause and reset your mind.

4. Eating: Plan time in your day to eat at a relaxed, slow pace to keep your digestive system at its best. Try to regularly consume fermented foods or take a high quality probiotic supplement.

5. Vitamin D: Vitamin D is important for both your physical and mental health. When you have low levels of vitamin D, it's been shown to contribute to an increased risk of depression.

- Contributed by Dr. Rok Morin

Your mental health is just as important as your physical health. Thinking well and keeping your emotions positive can help you make huge steps toward a healthier life! Thoughts come with ramifications in our lives. When we think healthy, positive, vibrant, energetic, and optimistic thoughts we end up with a physiology that's vibrant, energetic, active and adaptable.

Start your day with empowerment! Wake up every morning and nourish your body with positive, optimistic thoughts about your success and your abilities that day. It's a better practice to wake up in the morning thinking "this is going to be my best day ever" instead of waking up in the morning thinking about how hard your day is going to be. The worst way to start the day emotionally and physiologically is with an attitude of "this is going to be a rotten day!"

Dr. Rok Morin, who is one of the partners of the Chiropractic Vitality Centers of Maine and a co-developer of Learning Curves and the Legion of Chiropractic, had a brilliant solution for some for our practice members who hated Mondays. He had bumper stickers made that said, "I Love Mondays!" Whenever he heard one of our practice members say, "Ugh, it's Monday," he'd give them a bumper sticker and ask them to cancel or change that thought and replace it with, "Yeah, I Love Monday, or Tuesday, or Wednesday, or Thursday, or Friday!"

You get the point: if you set the tone of your body with positive, optimistic, healthy thoughts, you'll create a tone and an energy that will lead to better cellular reproduction, reduced cellular breakdown, greater adaptability to stress, and greater control of your health expression. Greater optimism in your mind will lead to a higher energy level, a higher energy level leads to a higher level of vibration, a higher level of vibration leads to better choices, better choices lead to better adaptability, and better adaptability ultimately leads to a higher expression of life.

Think Well is a very important framework for building a well-adjusted life. In fact, many books have been written on this subject alone. Let's be honest here, life is challenging, and it's normal to experience times where it gets the better of us! The key is to not get down on ourselves when we are in an emotional state of thinking that doesn't serve us.

The key is to become more conscious. When we become more conscious of how we're thinking, then we can start to catch ourselves with negative, disempowering thoughts. If we don't catch the thought, we'll catch the state it creates. With negative or disempowering thoughts, we'll feel diminished energy in our body and might find ourselves with a slumping posture, feeling defeated and/or incapable of overcoming the obstacles ahead.

The "cure" when you feel disempowered is to cancel those thoughts and replace them with thoughts of optimism, energy, hope, resolve, and confidence. When you practice this level of conscious connection to your thoughts and feelings, you'll find that you can purposefully create a change in the way your body feels and functions, and you'll see a shift in your life. After all, your thoughts become your beliefs, your beliefs dictate your actions, and your actions create your outcomes.

Whatever your current health status or what you want to accomplish as a future goal, nothing will take the place of your commitment and willingness to take the first step to get moving. If you're ready to create the health you desire and deserve, I would love to be your leader on the journey to "My Life Well-Adjusted."

Chapter 6

You Cannot Overcome a Sick Lifestyle

There are many myths that run wild in society, but when it comes to health and/or sickness, there are 2 that cause more apathy than most: 1) Genes are the most influential factor in the development of disease or infirmity in life, and 2) Full-scope chiropractic care is only useful for people in pain.

Let's begin to dissect these myths one at a time, starting with the genetics "false flag" of disease. Without question, this myth is FALSE! It's important to know with certainty that genetics is probably not holding you back from gaining and maintaining a high level of health, nor is it holding you hostage in a state of impending disease.

With 25 years of experience in the practice of true healthcare, combined with an interest in research focused primarily on human potential, I've learned that there is a more empowering truth. The truth regarding the influence of genetics on health is that it pales in power compared to the influence of lifestyle.

When you focus an educated investigation on the findings of genetics, health sciences, and human performance research, you get a very different picture than that of the studies done in the world of pharmacology and bioengineering. In real scientific studies aimed to seek the truth about health and human performance, you find that one's state of health or sickness is clearly and convincingly affected most dramatically through lifestyle. Pharma and bioengineering studies paint a picture that is wholly self-serving and designed to sell a paradigm that does not serve you well! The facts point out that lifestyle is a determinant factor 85% of the time and genetics plays a lesser 15% role.

Why is this such an important distinction to make, you might wonder? Simply put, you can exert control over your genetics even though you didn't choose your genes or your parents. Regardless of what genes you were designed by in utero, you have absolute control over your lifestyle, and therefore, you have a large degree of control of your genetic expression in life. In other words, if you are one of the 85% of humans that doesn't have a genetic predisposition for a particular disease, you have 100% control over your health status. If you are one of the 15% with a genetic code for a particular disorder, you still have more power than you might believe.

For me, and the thousands of practice and community members I share this with, this is a much more empowering truth to live by compared to the false flag of the predetermined genetic disease myth. The myth of genetics has been a convenient story for the merchants of sickness products and services (the fast food, chemical, and pharmaceutical industries, and the sick care system). In fact, this smoke and mirrors myth has kept those industries fat and happy for over a century.

I fully believe that no one desires to get or be sick, but for the sake of this line of thought, let's say for a minute that you desire to be sick. If you have a desire to be sick, you'd have to do nothing more than live the lifestyle of most Americans, and fully engage in the sick care system of disease treatment. If you were to do what most people unfortunately do, you would accomplish sickness with brilliant success. The average American lives a lifestyle devoid of healthy movement, with limited quantities of healthy food, large quantities of unhealthy food, the paradigm of a pill for every ill, and a lifestyle where pessimism, fear, and unconscious living is far more prevalent than optimism, hope, and conscious planning.

In this chapter, I want to help you "flip the script" and set the stage for a much more meaningful and manageable life of optimal health expression. In chapter 5, "Eat Well, Move Well, Think Well," we discussed 3 powerful aspects of lifestyle and defined how your thoughts and actions determine your health outcomes. Lifestyle is so much more powerful than genetics in the development of your health expression. It deserves to be thought about, planned, and implemented with absolute consciousness, with a crystal-clear vision of the outcomes you desire, and defined by a meaningful set of goals, achieved through purposeful actions. "You cannot overcome a sick lifestyle."

If you're still wondering, "What if I'm one of those unfortunate 15% that has bad genetics?", stay positive. The field of science called epigenetics gives us hope by proving that genetic predispositions are more like premonitions, not foregone conclusions of disease. We are finding that our genes can be and are affected by a positive expression and higher states of adaptability through purposeful action in our lifestyle. That my friend is cheer worthy!

Lifestyle is so powerful that you can't beat it if you try and you can't overcome it if you don't. If you wanted to be sick, but in your efforts you mistakenly did everything right, meaning you ate well, moved well, and thought well, in most cases, you would fail to achieve sickness. Now on the flip side, let's say you truly desired to be well, but in your efforts to be well, you ate unwell, you thought unwell, and you moved unwell. I am sad to tell you, you'd fail to achieve health. This bold and unwavering truth is actually self-evident and self-actualizing.

The power to create health and/or sickness is yours to control. Your health or sickness is the outcome of the way you live your life!

If we look at the rates of obesity, cancer, diabetes, heart disease, or any of the most common diseases in the United States, the statistics show a devastating and staggering story of unconscious living. It's obvious that no one would ever consciously desire to develop type 2 diabetes, no one would purposefully create heart disease, and certainly no one would for any reason wish to have cancer affect their lives or that of a loved one! If this is true, and I believe it is, then why do so many people in the United States and abroad end up with these major diseases? The answer as we see it through the field of epigenetics, biology, physiology, and health sciences is simple: lifestyle imbalance.

It may be hard to read this without it feeling like a statement of judgment or admonishment, but please stay with me and trust me, I do not share this information to judge or to convict. I am the last person that would say anyone deserves to experience sickness, disease or infirmity in their lives. In fact, I am the biggest champion of optimal well-being you will ever meet!

I have witnessed literally thousands of my practice members turn their life conditions from dis-ease to optimal ease through the recommendations I share, the care I provide, and by living the principles and practices of full-scope chiropractic care (Track 1) and the Success Triad (Track 2) of the "My Life Well-Adjusted" program. Please know with certainty that regardless of where you are starting, better health is an option in your life.

It is well established that lifestyle is predominantly responsible for our state of health or sickness. It really is that simple, and it all comes down to adaptability. I will say adaptability over and over and over, in fact, those who know me well say it's my favorite "drum to beat." My definition of adaptability is "the ability to meet and overcome the daily physical, chemical, and mental/emotional challenges in life." Adaptability is *the key* to successful, vibrant health.

The next myth that deserves to die a timely death is that full-scope chiropractic care is only useful for people who are in pain. This myth is perpetuated mostly due to a complete lack of understanding on 2 different but related fronts.

The first front is that most health care professionals and the general public don't understand what full-scope chiropractic care is, but they think they do. What this incongruence of understandings creates is a false belief that health care and sick care are the same, and that full-scope chiropractic is a sick care system. Full-scope chiropractic is not a sick care model, it is a health care model that cannot be fit into the sick care model and make sense.

Chiropractic is the proverbial square peg (health care) in the round hole (sick care). To be fair, in a program of full-scope chiropractic care, there is an initial short phase of care that is partially designed to help reduce symptoms of pain, stiffness, or inflammation, but that is merely the tip of the iceberg of what full-scope chiropractic care is designed to address. If pain is the tip of the iceberg, the real health benefits that full-scope chiropractic delivers is the mountain of ice you don't see under the water. It's the mountain of ice under the water that most physicians are not trained to look for or just don't see, that sinks the health of most patients in a sick care model.

Full-scope chiropractic care is different! If you were to come to my office or visit one of the "My Life Well-Adjusted" doctors, you would be educated on the difference between palliative care (symptom based) and full-scope chiropractic care (whole health based). Palliative care or sick care is short term, unidimensional, and narrow focused (pain care). Full-scope chiropractic care is long term, multidimensional, and has a wide focus (complete care).

Why most health care professionals and people in the general public get this wrong is because they have never been trained to think beyond the short term, unidimensional, and narrow focus of the sick care model. Most people that seek care in a sick care model do so for a particular symptom.

In the sick care model, the focus of the visit by the patient and the doctor is *the symptom*, so the treatment is prescribed to merely reduce the symptom, and that's all folks! In a full-scope chiropractic health care model, most people seek care for a particular symptom, just like in the sick care scenario above. But in the full-scope chiropractic office, the care delivered will be focused to detect and correct *the cause* of the symptom, not to merely treat or reduce it.

At Bangor Family Chiropractic, or any of the Chiropractic Vitality Centers of Maine, we only recommend care after we have all the facts, understand the complete cause of the problem, and have determined a solution. In a whole health model, the purpose of care is very different, and the process is much more detailed and complete. If getting well is the goal, the following steps must be taken to ensure success:

- A complete consultation to determine history and goals.

- A comprehensive examination, usually including x-rays, to assess the objective cause of the current condition, as well as ascertaining the subjective complaints of the member.

- A thorough report of findings to ensure a complete understanding of the condition and the means to correct the cause.

- A comprehensive care plan determined by the doctor and agreed upon by the practice member.

- Regular re-examinations to gauge progress and adjust methods.

The difference between the 2 models is profound and powerful! Palliative sick care is a single phase of care with a narrowly defined focus which addresses symptoms not the cause. At the end of a sick care phase of treatment the symptoms may be gone, but the condition is still there and getting worse without your awareness.

In the full-scope chiropractic model, which is a multi-phasic model, the care is delivered over a continuum where the symptoms are addressed (Phase I), the cause is corrected (Phase II) and health maintenance is monitored through regular wellness care to ensure long term optimal well-being (Phase III).

The most damaging effect of a short-term, single phase, narrow focused sick care model is what it does to the consumer. In the sick care model, the aim is to reduce the symptoms of a symptomatic person, not to get to the cause of the symptoms, so it is at best an incomplete model.

The complete sick care model looks like this: a sick and symptomatic person seeks care, care is delivered to reduce the symptoms, and patient leaves care expecting to be healthy. What really occurs is at the core of the devastating statistics we see in our health as a society. The true outcome of a sick care model is this: sick and symptomatic people are treated to reduce symptoms and are left a sick and asymptomatic person, as the cause was never detected and corrected. It is sure to get worse over time and escalate the need for intervention in the future.

The fact is that you cannot overcome a sick lifestyle, this is a time proven, irrefutable, and absolute truth. Consider type 2 diabetes for instance, which is a leading cause of severe, acute, and chronic sick care visits with lifelong medical needs, and devastating physical, financial, and social ramifications. Type 2 diabetes, heart disease, arthritis, and most cancers are not genetic conditions, but are born from lifestyle, and they are increasingly robbing our communities of resources.

When we live a sick lifestyle, we become dependent on a sick care system, and our sick care system is broken! Our sick care system of reactive care in the face of disease is such a disastrous paradigm that has failed us so badly, it's now the third leading cause of death, right behind cancer and heart disease. That's right, you read that properly. Our health care system as it's called is the third leading cause of death in the United States!

It's not the doctors, nurses, and other health professionals that are bad, or mean harm, or are poorly trained. It's the paradigm that is broken! We've come to believe that our supposed health care system will save us from sickness, but it won't. That belief numbs us to the reality of lifestyle. There is no pill that ever made someone healthy, no surgery that will correct the cause, and no medical intervention that will make you well.

The chart below is taken from the British Medical Journal and it makes the case for focusing on lifestyle and the need for safe, specific, and scientific, health care that is reliable and focused on causes not symptoms.

Death in the United States

Johns Hopkins University researchers estimate that medical error is now the third leading cause of death. Here's a ranking by yearly deaths.

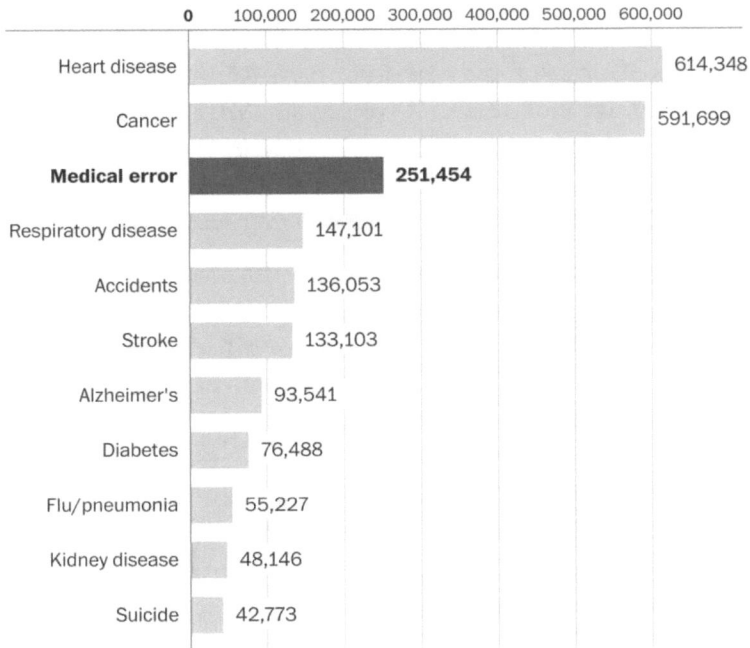

Cause	Deaths
Heart disease	614,348
Cancer	591,699
Medical error	**251,454**
Respiratory disease	147,101
Accidents	136,053
Stroke	133,103
Alzheimer's	93,541
Diabetes	76,488
Flu/pneumonia	55,227
Kidney disease	48,146
Suicide	42,773

Source: National Center for Health Statistics, BMJ   THE WASHINGTON POST

As I stated before, and you probably agree, no one desires to get or be sick. Unfortunately, it's not a desire to be sick that causes the level of sickness we see in society, but a lack of knowledge, forethought, planning, and the ability to make educated decisions. As a society, we've been brainwashed into being "comfortably numb" by the false promise that the sick care system supported by insurance coverage will rescue us. The question is not whether one desires to be sick. The question we need to begin asking ourselves is, "do I desire to be ultra-healthy?" Planning to depend on the safety net of our sick care system is an ideology that has major flaws and dire consequences for our future. IT SIMPLY DOESN'T WORK!

If you desire to be an optimal weight, to have optimal function of all systems, and have a healthy composition of lean muscle and healthy bone structure, it takes consistent and persistent effort. Without consistent, persistent, and conscious effort, you may find yourself following the prescription for sickness that we see showing up as generational life habits. We learn patterns of thought and action that are hard to bend or break if we aren't aware and purposefully dedicated to an ideal that serves us better.

To reinforce the concept of the power of focus on lifestyle, I'll use myself as an example. 10 years ago, I found myself so engrossed in caring for others that I wasn't caring for myself. As a result, my life was out of balance. I was busy in my practice working far too many hours and days each week. I was getting far too little sleep to be healthy. "I didn't have the time" (or so I thought) to engage in regular exercise. I wasn't thinking about food as nutritious fuel for life, so I'd grab breakfast or lunch on the run and eat dinner late.

I wasn't conscious of my thought patterns beyond the project I was working on. I was generally rolling with the punches of my professional life. I was successful in ways that didn't matter but I was failing in critical areas that did.

One day while reviewing photos from a seminar series I produced, I saw a picture of myself that told a truth that I'd been ignoring. I was 20 plus pounds overweight, or by body composition standards, I was 40 pounds overweight. It was obvious that my clothes didn't fit the way they used to. Although I wasn't tired, I looked exhausted!

As I did a little reflection on the reality of the moment, I realized that I felt generally unbalanced with my energy, stamina, and drive, and I was living a very unconscious existence. In that moment I decided that I was going to make the changes that would save my life. I was going to become the person I didn't see in that picture!

10 years later, I'm happier, healthier, more fit, and I have more balance in my personal and professional life than I would have if I hadn't taken action. Deciding to live a conscious and goal-oriented lifestyle, with a crystal-clear vision of what I wanted in each dimension of my life (physical, mental, social, financial, spiritual, professional, and emotional) allowed me to work smarter not harder.

What I found in my own personal journey was that when I focused on enhancing the quality of one dimension of life, the benefit bled into all the other dimensions of my life. In that moment, I began building a process of living that I call the Success Triad. The basis of the Success Triad (which I will discuss in-depth in later chapters) is Track 2 of the "My Life Well-Adjusted" journey. It's a whole life system of defining and designing the most balanced, compelling, and meaningful life possible in all dimensions.

When we take the time to evaluate our lives, we find that we are habitual beings, living habitual patterns, that perpetuate our current state and dictate our future if we let them. Of course, we all have areas of success in our personal and professional lives that we can and should be proud of. I'm not at all suggesting that we as individuals or as a race of humans are abject failures. I am, however, suggesting that if we define, design, and deploy a well-planned and purposeful path, we'll have even more great things to celebrate, and we'll create the life that most inspires us.

The current patterns in our lives come from our past, primarily from the influences of our Mothers, Fathers, Teachers, and Preachers (MFTP's), or in other words, the very people that shaped who we've become. Some of our patterns of thought and action are good and some not so good. Wouldn't you agree?

When I'm fortunate enough to work with my practice members to help them create a more vital life, I recommend that they keep the good and banish or replace the not so good. If you've learned optimism, keep it. If you've learned poor eating habits, replace them. If you grew up drinking soft drinks, replace them with water. If you aren't as active as you need to be to express high levels of health, set a goal that is achievable, and get moving. (More on SMART goal setting in chapter 8).

Our lifestyle of eating, moving, thinking, and the core ideologies that define how we live our lives are strongly influenced by the people we spend the most time with. These people are our mentors, role models, trusted advisors and the shapers of our current life outcomes, in ways we don't even realize.

The people we learned great habits from are the same people we learned not so great habits from. By evaluating our patterns, we can keep the great ones and replace the rest. It's important to give credit where credit is due, while at the same time understanding the need to assess and evaluate the ideas and influences that have shaped our world view.

I always make it a point to show gratitude to my MFTP's, but I'm careful to make sure that the ideas and actions I adopt serve my life purpose well. To add clarification to the concept of MFTPs, and to highlight the power we have to embrace the good and dismantle the bad, I'd like to share this article written by Dr. Rachel Fogarty of the Chiropractic Vitality Centers of Maine.

MFTP – Mother, Father, Teacher, Preacher

"MFTP refers to the idea that your current beliefs, ideas, concepts, actions and reactions to life's events have been developed by your adherence to the influences of your mother, father, teachers, and preachers. The current state of your life, whether it is good – meaning as you would dream it, or bad – meaning nightmarish, is largely based on your personal beliefs and actions. Thoughts create your beliefs, your beliefs create your actions, and your actions create your reality.

As a doctor, I get the opportunity to work with many people who have a variety of different conditions and/or issues affecting their health. The one common theme that is revealed in most of the cases that I see is that the condition or issues that caused the health crisis in the first place are based either in part, or as a whole, on lifestyle. The cause of the poor lifestyle choices is most usually due to the person making decisions that are based on misinformation or a total lack of information with which to guide their decision-making process.

Lack of information is usually easier to work with because it does not come loaded with bias and justification. Misinformation is much tougher to overcome. The reason for this is because the information came from a source that is trusted, valued, or has an honored place in our lives. It is sometimes easier for us to continue to believe than to face the reality that we may have developed a belief, action, and outcome that was wrong or hurtful. To admit to faulty thinking we may feel that we are in a way accusing our trusted advisors of misleading us or providing us with harmful information.

As a doctor of chiropractic, the advice I give my patients can be very different from the advice that my patients have received from their mothers, fathers, teachers, preachers, and in many instances, their other healthcare advisors. This is not to say that anybody is wrong or intentionally giving false and/or misleading information. It is more often a difference in perspective. Our perspective on life is heavily dependent on our past thinking and conditioned by the information we have been provided through our MFTP, the media, and/or other sources.

One way of making decisions in life is to make sure that you first look at what your personal bias is. Think about the ways you have dealt with similar situations in the past and look at the outcomes. If you are satisfied with the previous outcomes, then trust your conditioned thinking. If you did not achieve the desired outcome, re-examine your thinking and look for different ideas and approaches. Consult others and ask for their opinions and see if there is a different way of approaching the situation using a different thought pattern or approach. Some examples of these situations are the issues of weight loss, deteriorating health, retirement planning, career changes, parenting issues, etc.

If you are struggling with these issues and you have been searching the same data bank, meaning yourself, and approaching them with the same pattern of thought, meaning the thoughts you have been conditioned to believe from your MFTP, and getting the same unsatisfactory results time after time, don't be disheartened. Simply admit that you do not have the answers and ask for help. Talk to someone who has achieved success in that particular endeavor and try to understand how they may be looking at the issue differently and how that perspective may be the only difference between your failure and their success. It is very possible that this dialog may lead others to you with questions about some areas where you may excel where they are struggling.

We all have strengths and we all have weaknesses and in the end it is our past that reinforces both. To create strength where there was a weakness, we may have to shed our past thinking and replace it with a different pattern."

- Dr. Rachel Fogarty

In reality, what I'm suggesting is a process of consciously and critically evaluating what it is you want to create in your life and then adopting a new paradigm to help you achieve it. If you desire optimal health, vibrant well-being, and abundance in all dimensions of your life, I believe you can develop the ability to consciously build the framework of thoughts and actions that would allow you to have it. Full-scope chiropractic care and the "My Life Well-Adjusted" life planning and development program will help you achieve optimal health and well-being, vital adaptability to physical, chemical, mental/emotional stress, abundance of physical, intellectual, and emotional resources, and will increase the quality and quantity of your life.

I'd like to share a couple pieces of writing from 2 of my closest friends and colleagues that highlight 3 very necessary ingredients for change. Dr. Trevor Bevans is a friend and colleague that I've worked with in The Chiropractic Vitality Centers of Maine, and he shares a story about courage and conscious living. As health care professionals we recognize that change takes courage and a conscious choice to achieve it.

The Lifestyle Train

"Imagine you are on a train, a train that represents your life. Where is that train headed and how fast is it getting there? You were born, and one day you will leave this life. What's important is the direction you are headed in and the tracks you choose to travel.

Are the choices you make today moving you towards an extraordinary life of abundance and health, or are you traveling down the tracks of scarcity and dis-ease? Regardless of where you are headed, it is imperative that you recognize where you are, where you are going, and whether it is where you want to end up. Ignorance is not bliss if you want to live an extraordinary life. Where you will be ten years from now will be a result of the choices you make today and in the future.

I realize, of course, that there are things that happen to you, that are out of your control. It's how you choose to respond that will make all the difference. While doing a Tough Mudder last year in Vermont I heard about this guy, Noah Galloway, who wasn't like all the other Mudders out on the 10.2 mile course of harsh mountain terrain. You see, Noah is a 32 year old retired Army Sergeant who, on December 19, 2005, lost his left arm above the elbow and left leg above the knee in an Improvised Explosive Device (IED) attack in Yusafiah, Iraq. After this tragedy Noah fought through the depression he could have fallen victim to and chose to "inspire others by his actions, by training like a machine and demonstrating that challenges are meant to be conquered no matter how big they might be." The image of him running up "Everest" on his prosthetic leg with fellow Mudders there to assist is inspiring! He competes in other similar events with other "Wounded Warriors" and is a motivational speaker. Again, we can't always control what happens to us, only how we act in response.

Reflect on your life and health. Ask yourself, "Do I have strategies in place for meeting all the requirements for health?" There are 4 major requirements:

You must have a clear brain-body connection. Energy and information must be able to flow throughout your nerve system without interference. The best and only strategy for meeting this requirement is being checked regularly by a full-scope chiropractic practitioner.

You must be feeding yourself with whole foods that your body was designed to be fueled by.

You must be moving your body the way nature intended. Functional exercise programs that focus on improving mobility and strength through full ranges of human movement.

Finally, in order to live an extraordinary life you must live consciously. Through reflection and investigation into your beliefs, you can determine the truths that are motivating your actions. You must also discover your purpose and approach life with passion and positive self-esteem. As Hal Elrod says in his book *The Miracle Morning*, "Why is it that when a baby is born, we often refer to them as 'the miracle of life', but then go on to accept mediocrity for our own lives? Where along the way did we lose sight of the miracle *we* are living?" Your life is no accident and it's meant to be extraordinary.

It's easy to read and write about how to make your life extraordinary. In reality it takes work. It's worth it though and it gets easier with time. The most important thing to remember is that living a healthy lifestyle is a choice and you can only receive the benefits for as long as you choose to engage in life enhancing strategies.

Throughout life your train is either moving towards abundance and health or towards sickness and disease, never are we standing still! Like a train that can't stop on a dime and change directions, when you want to move your life and health in another direction it will take time to change course but time will go by either way. So, don't give up on healthy behaviors because change isn't happening fast enough. Apply the concepts you know to be true and persist.

A friend and former co-worker recently announced that she had finally reached her goal of losing 100 pounds! She didn't accomplish this overnight, she adopted life enhancing strategies and persisted. It has taken her 2 and a half years to accomplish what she has, and she's not stopping now because she realizes health is a journey not a destination.

Life is meant to be extraordinary. Live it!"

- Dr. Trevor Bevans

Dr. Rok Morin is one of the founding partners of The Chiropractic Vitality Center of Maine and the owner and leader of our team at Holland Chiropractic Wellness Center in Bath, Maine. In the article he wrote for the "Wellness News You Can Use" monthly newsletter he shares the concept of embracing fear as a useful empowerment tool for overcoming obstacles on your path to accomplishing your goals.

Fearless Living

"Fearless living, what a concept! I wanted to write this article this month because the idea of living fearlessly and banishing all fear, worry, doubt, insecurity, and uncertainty has become a very hot topic in the popular press these days. You hear about this concept on television shows like Oprah, you see whole sections of the book stores filled with books that profess that you can live fearlessly, you see articles in most self-help magazines almost monthly that suggest that it is the optimal height of living when you can throw caution and concern to the wind and live the "warrior way."

I believe that living fearlessly is impossible, and I contend that it is much more appropriate to live a life with less fear than to live a fearless life. It may sound to some like I am just changing the words around, but there is a profound difference between a life of less fear and a fearless life. The difference lies in the depth, breadth, and width of our awareness. Living with less fear takes a level of consciousness that does not exist with living a fearless life. It requires that we become students of our past and masters of our futures. Living with less fear is a much more courageous way to live life because it demands that we become willing to face our past experiences and the patterns of belief that we have cultivated over the years into strong belief patterns and re-examine them in a framework of reality.

We have all heard the acronym for fear as being False/Evidence/Appearing/Real and that is why living fearlessly is living without conscious awareness; it actually means that we ignore our past and act in a way that is false or misleading to our belief patterns. Living fearlessly does nothing to rewire those false beliefs so they will naturally live on to challenge us in the future. Living with less fear means that we hold fear as a reality, we recognize it and we define its origins and challenge its hold on us. Living with less fear is a process that allows us to develop real clarity, and a new set of evidence, and that clarity lifts us up with heightened strength and power which naturally leads to greater freedom. Freedom is the catalyst to change, and changing your past fears to new realities is what it takes to master living with less fear and greater opportunity.

So, begin today. Challenge your fears, dig into the past and evaluate the false evidence that created them and commit to make new agreements with yourself that will create new beliefs and banish the need to act on disempowered false patterns of thinking that have held you back. Forget living fearlessly and begin the journey of awareness and clarity and live with less fear today!"

- Dr. Rok Morin

Do you want to be fully active and engaged in the outcome of your life? If you do, "My Life Well-Adjusted" is exactly the program for you! With full-scope chiropractic care you will have the adaptability to overcome the physical, chemical, and mental/emotional stresses of life, and with the "My Life Well-Adjusted" program you will be able to make values-based, vision-oriented, and purposeful actions to live your ideal life.

If you're ready to take the leap for life, I'd like to be your coach and leader on your journey to a life well-adjusted, *A Life Worth Living*.

You cannot overcome a sick lifestyle, but you can build an extraordinary one!

Chapter 7

What is Wellness?

Wellness is a term or concept that is used so often by people in almost every industry to describe completely different things. At best it's overused, and at worst it's been diminished to a point where it's ignored by practically everyone. It's thrown around by sick care providers, health care providers, pharmacies, gyms, supplement companies, veterinarians, insurance companies, and just about everyone that provides any product or service to the public. Wellness is not a product or any one action. Wellness is an outcome, and it's multidimensional.

The best definition of wellness, in my opinion, is from the World Health Organization, which states the following: "Wellness is an active process of becoming aware of and making choices towards a healthy and fulfilling life. Wellness is a state of complete physical, mental, and social well-being, and not merely the absence of disease or infirmity."

I like this description and definition because it conveys the truth about wellness. Wellness is a process, not an event. You can't "take" wellness, but instead you create wellness. Most importantly, being well is not about how you feel, it's about how you function in all dimensions of life. Wellness is a state of being where you have balance, homeostasis, critical thinking, purposeful action and great functional outcomes. In other words, it's an accumulation of thoughts and actions. It's more than being free of illness, it's a dynamic process of change and growth.

The National Wellness Institute defines wellness as follows: "Wellness is conscious, as in you're making a decision, you're creating a plan, a conscious self-directed and evolving process of achieving full potential." It goes further, defining wellness in 6 dimensions: "Wellness is multidimensional and wholistic, encompassing lifestyle, mental and spiritual well-being, and the environment. Wellness is positive and affirming."

The creation of the "My Life Well-Adjusted" program of wellness development was cultivated from the accumulated knowledge and skill I've developed working with many thousands of practice members over 25 years of active practice. I've come to know with absolute certainty that the development of wellness in life is a multidimensional process.

In the "My Life Well-Adjusted" wellness development model we focus on 2 tracks that run parallel and work in harmony:

Track 1: Physical and physiological well-being is addressed through full-scope chiropractic care. In Track 1 we reconnect the brain and the body to allow for the dynamic adaptability and self-regulation that is needed to fully express wellness.

Track 2: A whole life planning and development program is designed around the Success Triad training model of Be Genuine, See Clearly, Act Purposefully. The Success Triad system helps our practice members create a fully conscious system to maximize wellness in 7 dimensions of life: physical, mental, social, financial, spiritual, professional, and emotional.

Wellness is not just a catch phrase, it's not an event, and it's not something anyone can give you or prescribe for you. It's more than a lack of sickness, it's the accumulation of good inputs over a period of time and the outcome those actions create.

If you recall from chapter 4, we covered the difference between light and dark as an analogy to health/ease and sickness/dis-ease. I'd like to refresh that understanding now regarding this bigger and more comprehensive state of wellness.

Health is normally considered in a single dimension, whereas wellness is multidimensional and much more comprehensive in its meaning. Remember this: dark or dis-ease is an absence, and health is a presence. Ease is a state of abundance and dis-ease is a state of lack or absence.

Health as it pertains to any individual dimension can be achieved, but if it's not present in every dimension of life, it will ultimately affect all dimensions and interfere with achieving a state of wellness as a whole. Wellness is all encompassing, multidimensional, and it takes a defined and designed focus on conscious living with consistent and persistent thoughts and actions to gain, regain and maintain.

I absolutely love providing care and coaching in the "My Life Well-Adjusted" model of multidimensional wellness development because it changes lives on a much deeper level than the models I used earlier in my career. Even though I was able to help a ton of people improve their health in the physical and physiological dimension with my earlier practice model of full-scope chiropractic care (Track 1), adding the Whole life Planning and

Development training of the Success Triad (Track 2) has taken the results for my practice members to new heights.

The practice of the "My Life Well-Adjusted" program has allowed my practice members to thrive at much high levels because it allows us to address all 7 dimensions of life in a unified approach.

I willfully admit that achieving wellness in the "My Life Well-Adjusted" model is not a walk in the park. It can be a challenge for people to choose to initiate wellness in their lives, and therefore it may not be right for everyone. Becoming well is not easy or quick, and becoming well is not what everyone wants, but it is what some people want, and those are the people I attract to my practice. I'm okay with being the doctor that specializes my care towards those looking for the highest quality results in life. I love seeing the outcomes my practice members achieve, it's exhilarating to see the proverbial "light come on" for my members!

Let me be clear, most people visit me initially looking for something much less involved than creating wellness in their lives! That's okay. Some want pain relief, others want a solution to their headaches, and some are looking to regain their active lifestyle so they can enjoy their retirement.

Regardless of *why* someone comes to me, they usually realize they are in exactly the right place. I help many people that want to focus specifically on the physical and physiological aspects of health, and that is where full-scope chiropractic shines. But some want a more comprehensive, whole life approach, and that's where the "My Life Well-Adjusted" approach to total wellness fits the bill.

The most important aspect of a successful relationship with your care provider is defining and designing the best outcomes possible for you (the practice member) and them (the provider). I have one non-negotiable standard that I refuse to bend when it comes to my obligation and responsibility when starting the provider/member relationship: I must be given the opportunity to make optimal recommendations for care based on the findings of my consultation and exam.

I don't have the authority to dictate whether someone accepts my care, and wouldn't want it, but I do maintain the right to accept or reject a person from membership to my office. (Very few people are rejected once we complete our discovery together). I've found that having high practice standards is essential to achieve high outcomes and it serves everyone well. In the most basic terms, when it comes to my professional life, "I am in it to win it" for my practice members. There should be no other way!

Wellness is the total accumulation of the inputs from all dimensions of life, including, but not limited to, the thoughts we think, the foods we choose to eat or not eat, the way we move our bodies, and the quality and quantity of information that passes from body to brain and brain to body. Wellness shows up when we have an uninterrupted expression of the constructive and creative intelligence that made the body (innate intelligence).

The intelligence that coordinates the external world we live in is called universal intelligence. Innate intelligence is constructive, whereas universal intelligence is destructive by nature. Innate intelligence is the internal force that is required to meet and manage the destructive external force of nature known as stress. There is stress in every moment of every day of our lives. We would not and could not exist without universal force, and we would not and could not live without innate forces to adapt to universal forces.

Universal force/stress is necessary for the existence of life, but if we lack the ability to adapt to it, we lose the ability to self-regulate and coordinate the reactions and responses to equalize its influence. That lack of adaptability to universal force in called dis-ease. Dis-ease left undetected and uncorrected will eventually express itself as full-blown disease. This weakened state of dis-ease is the state of asymptomatic sickness that we talked about in chapter 6, and it's the usual outcome of the conventional sick care model.

When we have an interruption in the full expression of innate intelligence, we lack the potential to overcome universal forces, and that causes a continuous and unrelenting break down of tissue, leading to reduced ability to self-regulate, and ultimately the loss of the ability to self-heal.

"Wellness is an optimal state of physical, mental, and social wellbeing, not merely the absence of disease or infirmity."

- World Health Organization

Let's consider a very real scenario that plays itself out millions of times every year in the United States, and hundreds of millions of times across the globe. I'll use myself in this scenario so as not to offend anyone.

I'm cruising along in my busy life, living fairly unconsciously, without a clearly designed and defined health or life plan. Suddenly, I have a health crisis of some magnitude, large or small. In this fictitious account of life, let's assume I've never given much thought to the need to start my day with conscious preparation or a consistent plan to ensure my energy, emotion, and vision align to create the day I want most.

On this day, like most days, I jump out of bed with no clear preparation or plan for my day. I just start getting stuff done! I scurry around to make sure the kids have everything they need to get out of the house on time (but something didn't make it to the car). I hurry to drop off the kids on time (because I am responsible). I may have to pick up the dry cleaning before work (because I have no clean shirts). I have to stop at the gas station (because I chose not to the night before). Now I'm potentially late for work, but I haven't eaten and I need coffee! Does this sound familiar? Sure it does!

Now, extrapolate this out in 7 dimensions of life and you can easily understand where all dimensions are interconnected and affected by our thoughts, actions, and outcomes in any dimension. In this too often true account of life scenario, my life doesn't implode, as I've gone to work every day like I'm supposed to. I've been in a perpetual rush but I still get my work done. My day ends later than I hoped, but I figure I can catch up on sleep tomorrow night, and I know (fingers crossed) that everything will get better because the weekend is coming, and I will get a break!

Too often and for too long, this is the "hamster wheel" of life for too many of us. It's no wonder we eventually end up feeling less balanced, more stiff, uninspired, and overwhelmed. Worst of all in this fictitious scenario, with all this stress, I've never made regular spinal and neurological care with a full-scope chiropractor a priority, so it has a greater impact on my life than it would otherwise! The difference between this scenario and a scenario where I eat, think, and move consciously and consistently well with a designed and defined plan shows up in the outcomes.

If you were the author of the story above, how would you write the ending? It would probably end with me falling behind and feeling perpetually frazzled, right? It may include a chapter about perpetual loss of energy, feeling down and tired. I may even begin giving up certain activities because I don't have the time or the physical well-being to do them any longer. I "pay" with stiffness, tension in my muscles, and a couple of days of pain when I do them. If this is the body of the story of life, how does it end? I GET SICK.

There are many names we give that state of sickness:

- Diabetes
- Heart disease
- Cancer
- Migraines
- Fibromyalgia
- Chronic fatigue syndrome
- Tendonitis
- Neck pain
- Back pain
- Arthritis
- Nervous breakdown
- Psoriasis
- Heartburn
- Constipation

And the list goes on.

Due to our training and the propaganda of the "better health through better chemistry" model, what do we do? We reach for a cure to the symptom or a treatment for the condition as we understand it. We may seek an over the counter remedy, like an antacid for heartburn (heartburn is not an antacid deficiency), or an aspirin for our headache (headaches are not an aspirin deficiency), or ibuprofen for our neck pain (pain is not an ibuprofen deficiency). Or we may go to the doctor where we'll most likely be treated with stronger prescription strength pills to "really get the job done!"

Drugs work at reducing symptoms. They can interfere with inflammation, but who says inflammation should be interfered with? They are culturally considered relatively safe. But when it comes to critical thinking in the direction of creating healthy conditions for life, we know that at best they are a panacea, and at worst they make the underlying condition much worse, and they make the effects of the imbalance many times more damaging.

I'll say it again: the only way to create health is to face life with a well-designed and purposefully defined set of goals and actions that will enhance the body's ability to adapt to stress, self-regulate and self-heal. In other words, we cannot expect to live life on the terms of the above scenario and expect anything other than a diminished state of health where sickness takes root.

Our sick care system, based on the premise of the better health through better chemistry paradigm, is a dismal failure, and as a society we are paying the price. If you end up with a sore throat or infection and you take an antibiotic, it may kill the infecting bacteria, but it will not correct the reason you were susceptible in the first place.

An antibiotic does not fight off infection, it kills the invading bacteria, highjacks your immune response, and leaves you more susceptible to infection in the future. Our well-designed system of trained thinking causes us to ignore the conditions that cause sickness in exchange for the feeling of being well. But remember, you cannot get health by taking sickness away.

The best answer to living a life of balanced wellness is to understand what wellness is. If we desire to be truly well, we have to move away from the concept of "if I feel good I must be healthy, if I feel bad I must be sick." We need to move away from this allopathic, reactive responsive pattern of sick care and decide once and for all to choose patterns of thought and action that serve us. It's absolutely possible to create a state of health and wellness prosperity in your life, and you deserve it!

Health and wellness prosperity is not a monetary concept, it's a concept of resources. We create health and wellness resources through thoughts, actions, and outcomes. The key missing component of achieving optimal well-being in our society is our lack of knowledge and/or disregard of the relationship between the structure of the body and the function of the nervous system. When there is disfunction or imbalance in the body it causes the nervous system to lose its ability to adapt to stress effectively, self-regulate efficiently and overcome the challenges that move us toward sickness and disease.

Infection doesn't happen due to the presence of bacteria, it happens due to the absence of proper immunological responses. Spinal disease is not the presence of degeneration, it is the lack of proper joint motion, neurological balance, proper circulation, cellular health, and motor adaptation. The only way to avoid sickness is to live a well-designed and defined lifestyle that is crafted with WELLNESS in mind.

Wellness is a process of expressing full adaptation to life, not merely removing compensation or sickness and dis-ease. Wellness is the accumulation of healthy self-regulation and self-healing that happens when you have a balanced lifestyle and a focus on caring for your health instead of treating sickness.

Chapter 8

The Success Triad

As a healthcare provider, I'm given the opportunity to work with people of all ages, sizes, educations, religions, and lifestyles. In the many years that I've practiced, I've come to believe a couple fundamental truths:

- People do not plan their health.
- People do not plan their sickness.

Pretty profound, isn't it? The reasons there is little to no planning in either direction is simple:

- Life is busy and we get caught up in the every-day activities of getting by or "getting it done!"
- There is little to no training or educational opportunities to help us learn how or why to define or design a purposeful life.
- It is difficult to take on the purposeful planning of life when it is not part of our paradigm or world view. (This is a symptom of the 2 reasons above).

In consultation with practice members over the years, I've witnessed far too many people trying to figure out what or where they went wrong with their health, and in many cases, wishing they could do some of it over! The answer is the same for everyone: there is no doing it over, but there is a restart button and that is empowering!

I have the distinct advantage of having enough experience to put fears to rest and share an inspired and empowering new concept for my members. Even though every practice member I have worked with is unique in many ways, the condition most people are in when I get the chance to consult with them is not unique. The state of health at any given stage of life, in any dimension of life, is predictable and easily understood if you understand the key areas of health development and disease prevention.

I'm glad to be able to pass on the gift of my education and practice experience to those who desire defined, designed, and implemented strategies to regain and maintain wellness in their lives. As I've stated before, the bulk of my professional life has been focused exclusively in the physical and physiological realm of life using full-scope chiropractic care as a primary model of care.

My career has been unbelievably rewarding, and an amazing journey which I've loved! As rewarding as it's been to serve so many people in the past using full-scope chiropractic, I'm very excited about the future, and the addition of the whole life planning and development program of "My Life Well-Adjusted!"

I couldn't have known where the journey of my 25 years of providing successful outcomes would lead if I hadn't defined and designed my personal and professional life the way I have. I didn't come naturally to the idea of life planning, but it was through years of coaching, mentorship, and surrounding myself with great thinkers that has made all the difference.

At Bangor Family Chiropractic, I'll be implementing 2 different tracks of care that will lead to success for each individual practice member. The track that fits best will depend on the desired outcome for each member. I've developed the 2-track system of full-scope chiropractic

(Track 1) and whole life planning and development (Track 2) as a result of working with some of the best and brightest minds in the healthcare and personal development field. I'm very clear in my desired approach of providing care and I feel "My Life Well-Adjusted" will allow me to serve my practice members at the highest level in my new community!

Track 2 of the "My Life Well-Adjusted" program of care is the whole life planning and development phase of care known as the Success Triad. The Success Triad is a pattern of consciously and confidently living a life with the express intent of creating a balanced, exciting, meaningful, and rewarding life. Or as our graduates say, *A Life Worth Living*!

A well-adjusted life is a life that is balanced in 7 critical dimensions, which creates meaningful outcomes that are predictable, rewarding, empowering, and satisfying! Please do not take this to mean that I'm somehow suggesting your life is less GREAT than it should be! The inspiration to create the "My Life Well-Adjusted" program is the culmination of working with thousands of practice members and clients over several decades. It's the expression of my sense of responsibility to help those who are ready to create the lives they desire and deserve.

It's been my experience that most of the symptoms of imbalance in people's lives share a common cause. Most of the imbalance, disharmony, and dis-ease, which shows up as a failure to build the life most people want, is caused by a lack of purpose, clarity, planning, and implementation. In other words, a conscious and well-designed path that is measurable and achievable. Simply stated, the Success Triad of **Be Genuine, See Clearly, Act Purposefully** is the perfect order to build a life that is balanced in all dimensions.

Be Genuine refers to who you are from a core values perspective. Living each day with a conscious foundation of core values that interweaves with your actions, will truly allow you to build your best life!

See Clearly is the step that allows you to be creative, be courageous, and be clear on the picture of your life that most inspires you. In essence, this step becomes your compass.

Act Purposefully is the final skill of the Success Triad for a reason. In this step you begin to take purposeful action that will allow you to consciously define, design, and most importantly, accomplish the goals and outcomes you desire most in life.

The first requirement to developing your optimal life is to believe that you deserve an optimal life. I believe you do. Do you?

Without exception, everyone I've ever talked to in my practice or in life in general wants to be successful. Not everyone has the same idea of what success means or looks like, but everyone wants to be successful. You might say there are many ways to gauge success, but for this moment, let's just say it means that you can trust that the time, energy, emotion, and money you commit to a project or a process will lead to the outcomes you most desire. It doesn't matter whether we're evaluating success from a physical standpoint, in personal or business relationships, financial statements, careers, or our overall health and well-being - we all want to know that our contributions are fulfilling a need, want, or desire for ourselves and most likely others.

In my career as a health care provider, I most often see people who have an unmet or unfulfilled need in the physical dimension of their lives, and a vast, overwhelming sense that there must be something different they could or should be doing, or should have done, to improve their health and well-being. Fortunately, when we do a complete consultation and evaluation of their current needs and their future health desires, we find that the cause (more often than not) is a lack of clarity in thought and action.

The "cure" is easy: understand what it is that you value, become knowledgeable about it, create a crystal clear vision of what you want, and be proactive in the quest for health, instead of continuing to be reactive in the treatment of disease.

The whole life planning and development track, in combination with the full-scope chiropractic track of the "My Life Well-Adjusted" program of care is designed to be a conscious and proactive program in a vitalistic and wholistic healthcare paradigm. I try to make this distinction very clear from the first conversation I have with prospective practice members, as it is a very different proposition than the standard sick care offerings.

The good news for nearly everyone I encounter in my practice is that the current state of their physical, mental, social, financial, spiritual, professional, and emotional lives, whether in a crisis state or just heading in the wrong direction, is reversible. Barring irreversible organic damage caused by extreme physical, chemical, or emotional trauma, most of society's illnesses are caused by a state of confusion which leads to inappropriate or ineffective lifestyle choices. The Success Triad is simple but powerful and it can be learned and implemented by anyone.

To achieve success in any and all areas of life, you must know what your values are and what you value the most.

The first action step in the Success Triad is the process of defining the key or core values that define why you do what you do. Your values define your purpose and help you establish your "Why." There is a saying in the personal development field that sums up the importance of getting clear on your core values very succinctly: "No Why, No Comply." What this means in real terms is that regardless of what you want, you will not attain it unless you attach a strong and compelling "Why" to it.

Your "Why" is the spark, the fuel, and reason to take you from awareness to action with full and unfettered resilience. Understanding your core values will allow you to move from awareness to purposeful action with confidence, direction, and success. Having well-defined and deeply conscious core values is what it takes to **Be Genuine**. To **Be Genuine** is to be empowered, and empowerment is necessary to build your well-adjusted life.

The next important step in the Success Triad is the process of developing a crystal clear vision of what you want to achieve or what you want to have "come into being" for yourself and/or others. In the life planning and development track of the "My Life Well-Adjusted" program, we call this the **See Clearly** state of goal setting and success.

Just as our core values are the compass, our vision is the X that marks the spot on our roadmap of life. The "Why" is important to get us started and allows us to stay engaged in meaningful action. The vision of where we're going and/or what we desire to create is essential to making sure we use our purposeful action in a direction that matters. In creating a more fulfilling and meaningful life, it's very important to use our time, energy, emotion, and resources as efficiently and effectively as possible so we don't end up overwhelmed or underachieved.

Having a crystal clear and compelling direction creates continuity and confidence on our journey. A nice Sunday drive in the country is a fun way to pass the time, but it is not directed with any specific and clear expectations or outcomes. We can't live every day of our life journey like a Sunday drive if we want to end up at a destination that is amazing!

In the **See Clearly** phase of the Success Triad we work as a team to create an inspiring, compelling, and crystal clear vision statement for the 7 dimensions of your life. It's this definition that will allow you to be directed in thought and action along the journey to your expected goal or defined outcome - an outcome that happens on purpose, not by chance!

Before I detail the final phase of the Success Triad known as **Act Purposefully**, I would like to share a very SMART concept of goal setting that my partner Dr. Tim Coffin shares with our practice members at Slocum Chiropractic Wellness Center in Brunswick, Maine.

Goal Setting the SMART way

"As you start on your journey to optimal health and the freedom to live without fear of dis-ease, I want to share this goal setting outline with you to help ensure you succeed. It is important to remember that for goals to be attainable (in this case, overcoming your health challenges or better yet, achieve optimal well-being), you need to write them down and read them regularly. New habits and the goals they allow you to achieve must be a part of your daily conscious thought for a minimum of 90 days before they become a subconscious activity or actionable outcome.

An effective guideline for setting goals is the SMART acronym. What the SMART goal setting guidelines actually mean is that your goals should be:

Specific, **Measurable**, **Attainable**, **Rewarding**, and **Timely**. When any of these steps are missing, the odds that your goals are achieved will drop substantially. Why? The key force that either drives you towards your goals or holds you back is your subconscious mind. These goal setting guidelines are the necessary criteria for your subconscious mind to accept your goals and start working for you, otherwise it will work hard to keep you in the comfort zone of your present conditions and old habits. Let's take the SMART guidelines and expand more specifically on their meaning.

Specific

With a specific goal you can clearly see what it is you want to achieve, and you have specific standards for that achievement. In making your goals specific it is important that you actually write them down, review them regularly, and revise them when appropriate. Goals must be written, reviewed, and revised to materialize! This step of the process is crucial in all goal setting guidelines. The more specific your goal is, the more realistic your success is, and the shorter the path to achievement. When you work on making your goal specific, you program your subconscious mind to work for you. When your subconscious mind is focused on a target, your thoughts and actions will lead you to your goal instead of pointing at the obstacles.

Measurable

For a goal to be measurable you must have a standard you can use to gauge your progress, and some specific criteria that will tell you when you must consider revising the goal, or if you have met it completely. Feeling the progress is very important for you to stay motivated and enjoy the process of achieving the goal. I will add one little caveat to this phase of the goal setting and achievement plan: some would say that it serves us best to increase our goal before we meet it to keep us pushing for higher heights, and I would agree.

Attainable

An attainable goal is a goal for which you see a realistic path to achievement, and reasonable odds that you will get there. This does not mean that the lower you aim the more likely you will be to reach success. It may actually be the opposite. My favorite quote on goal setting is by Michelangelo Buonarroti where he states: "The greater danger for most of us lies not in setting our aim too high and falling short; but in setting our aim too low, and achieving our mark." It is well known that the goals that work best have a challenge in them. The best goals are as ambitious as possible, but still reachable. When they are a stretch, they will give you more motivation and a greater sense of achievement when you succeed.

Rewarding

A goal is rewarding when you have clear reasons why you want to achieve it. Remember, "No Why, No Comply!" This is why your goals must be your goals and not someone else's concept or vision. It is best to have your specific reasons for reaching your goals and the expected rewards in writing, if possible with some visual pictures. Having a "goal board" or a "vision map" will help you imagine how you will feel when the goal is finally reached, and it will corral your creative energy along your journey. This step in the reward component of goal setting will help if you ever get stuck and don't feel motivated enough. (Trust me, there will be those moments). Having a compelling reason to stay motivated and on track is a very powerful, practical technique for getting through difficult moments and coming out a winner.

Timely

The fifth and final requirement of the SMART goal setting guidelines is also very important for your subconscious mind to set your achievement actions on target. Your goals should have a specific time limit or target date for achievement. Setting the deadline will protect you from paying a higher price than necessary to achieve them. Setting a firm timeline for achieving your goal will allow you to use every moment of your days, weeks, and months moving toward your target with efficiency. The last really important aspect of setting a specific timeline is to ensure you protect your vision of success from the sabotaging elements of procrastination and perfectionism.

Now that you know your guidelines for setting SMART goals, go out there and get what you have been waiting for, and have confidence that you will achieve it!"

- Dr. Tim Coffin

The last step in defining, designing, and implementing the Success Triad is to create the framework that will allow you to act in a way that directs your thought, actions, energy and enthusiasm in alignment with your values and your vision. This phase or step of the whole life planning and development track of "My Life Well-Adjusted" is known as the **Act Purposefully** phase.

If you want to exert a meaningful level of control on the ultimate outcomes of your life journey, it's not enough to merely go with the flow of life's twists and turns in a reactionary manner. Life must be lived purposefully. We only get one shot at this journey, so we might as well create the life we desire most instead of taking whatever we get by default.

The difference between living the "My Life Well-Adjusted" lifestyle and a reactionary one is measured by outcomes. If you want to have real direction, certainty, and the clarity to know you are on the right path and/or you desire to have more control or greater freedom, then you must engage the power of planning and conscious living. I'll go back to an earlier premise: "I have never met anyone that planned to create a state of lack in life, but I have met many that wished they had planned a state of abundance."

I desire to help you achieve *your* best possible life, and I know you can, as I have a lot of experience seeing people just like you transform their lives every day in my practice. I know you can create anything you want! If you're reading this and feel you are not getting the results you want in any of the 7 dimensions of your life (physical, mental, social, financial, spiritual, professional, and emotional), there is a way to change course and build the life you dream of!

If you don't know how to make that change, you are not alone! Unfortunately, in our busy world of teaching the fundamentals of math, English, science, and social studies, we've failed to educate and empower the knowledge of lifestyle development in youth.

If you're ready to make the conscious changes that will allow you to create what you desire most and deserve completely, but you don't know how to get it done, reach out to schedule your comprehensive health evaluation and your life planning and development consultation today.

If it sounds hard, IT IS. BUT YOU ARE WORTH THE EFFORT! If you question whether you can do it or not, YOU CAN. If you wonder if it is too late, IT IS NOT. If you question whether it is worth the effort, IT IS!

To create the life most people only dream of, you must live the **Be Genuine**, **See Clearly**, and **Act Purposefully** lifestyle to get it!

Chapter 9

Your Life Well-Adjusted –

Define, Design, Implement

Have you ever heard of the term "advanced citizenry?" Chances are, if you haven't heard the term, you know people in your community or your life that stand out as advanced citizens. They are the people whom everyone knows, they are the people whom everyone respects, they are the people whom other people turn to for information and services when they are in need. They are the people who, through their involvement in your community, have built a reputation of **trust,** and stand out as **valuable** contributors to the well-being of those they serve and/or those that depend on them.

They may be business leaders, politicians, teachers, coaches, or YOU. They may be involved with the ministry, doing mission work, or they may have started a community enrichment program for empowering citizens to create meaningful change. They may be the chief of police or head of the fire department, or they may be a mother or a father who cares about the neighborhood they live in. They are seen as cornerstones of our communities and they serve at a higher level than most.

To become an advanced citizen in your community, family, business or organization, and in your own life, you must develop the characteristics that all advanced citizens have in common.

In this chapter, I'll lay out the framework of the whole life planning and development work of Track 2 in the "My Life Well Adjusted" journey. I hesitated on whether to add this chapter initially, as I've found that few people can work this process successfully without a coach and a captain, for the reasons I highlighted in the previous chapter.

The reason it's difficult to accomplish this work independently is simple: without a coach who is objective and free of judgement, it can be difficult or nearly impossible to get past the subjective thoughts and actions that have become conditioned in your life. Your unique and deeply ingrained life experiences have shaped your paradigm, and in most cases, are hardwired into your thoughts, beliefs, and actions.

After many shifts in my thinking and consulting with practice members who have gained the full perspective of the impact of this model, I decided to add it with this caveat: I believe you can build the life of your dreams, but I feel strongly that life is not a solo journey. It takes a team, and often requires good coaching, mentoring, counseling, and compassionate care to create.

If you feel this effort is worthy and you decide that it is time for you to move into the planning and development of your ideal life, I beg you to allow me and/or one of my colleagues to assist you. I ask you to do this because I know it's not an easy task, although it is worth it, and I want to do my best to help ensure you get what you deserve from your worthy efforts.

When we break down our personal and professional lives, we have 3 major components or premises we need to clarify for us to be fully engaged and ultimately successful. These 3 components are **vision**, **mission**, and **purpose**. I'll define them in a very simple but empowering way for you to ensure accuracy and confidence on your journey.

Our Purpose is the "Why" (Be Genuine)

One of the first steps I guide my practice members through in Track 2 of the "My Life Well-Adjusted" journey is the initial values discovery process. In this activity, we begin by looking at the group of core values that have proven to be the most powerful and common when looking at global ethics research. As a primer to dig deeper and define them more clearly, I help my members to begin to write how these 7 core values have affected their lives in the past, and how they have shaped their outcomes in this moment.

As you read this, don't overthink this step, as it's the very beginning of a journey, not the end, and our conditioning will cause us to get stuck in the unfamiliar. One hint I would give, as I'm not there to guide and coach you, at least not yet, (fingers crossed in anticipation of being asked), is to use a piece of paper to "mind map" this, to see what comes off the top of your mind, instead of digging too deep into the recesses. There will be a time for digging deep and more thoughtful discernment later.

The following 7 listed values are not the only values that interact with your daily life, and these aren't meant to be the sole basis of your work on defining your purpose; however, they are the core values shared by most, therefore they make for a good starting point.

1. Responsibility: When you think of responsibility, what does that mean?

_____
_____
_____
_____
_____

2. Courage: Are there times when you have been challenged to act, speak out, or stand your ground? Where does your courage come from and how can you access it when needed?

_____
_____
_____
_____
_____

3. Respect: How does respect interface most often in your personal life, in "respect" to who you are as an individual or in other dimensions?

_____
_____
_____
_____
_____

4. Empathy: How does empathy impact your life and the lives of others in your circle of influence? How do you want it to contribute in the future?

_____
_____
_____
_____
_____

5. Justice: When faced with a dilemma, how important is it to you to see or create an outcome that feels just? Why is this important to you?

_____
_____
_____
_____
_____

6. Integrity: Absolute integrity is often talked about, a principle that most agree to be good, and a standard that can be difficult to adhere to. Describe the importance of integrity in your life.

_____
_____
_____
_____
_____

7. Discipline: How does discipline shape your life? Do you consider it an absolute value, a standard that you desire to consistently uphold, or something you struggle with but want to master?

_____

_____

_____

_____

_____

I've included these 7 core values for you to consider specifically, as they are the values that The Institute for Global Ethics found to be high order values, consistent on a global scale, regardless of race, ethnicity, gender, age, economic standing, religious affiliation, or geographic region of study.

After reading them, and writing your answers to the above questions, which of these particular values seem to be most in alignment with your world view, or seem to be primary drivers in your life? It's important to know that there is no need to be concerned about getting this "right" initially. You'll see as we go forward that your core values interact and interweave with your thoughts, actions, and outcomes with fluidity.

The important aspect of this values assessment work is to bring your "Why" to the forefront of your conscious evaluation in moments of meaning in life. In moments of brilliant power and clarity, it is your core values that are forefront and present and in moments of uncertainty, where you lack a sense of power or determination, it is your core values that are missing from the equation.

The activity above is the start of an evolving process of self-awareness and self-discovery, and should by no means be the final act in your assessment of the values that drive the outcomes of your life. You will, however, start to become more aware of the "Why" that will become a primary driver in the development of power and purpose for your future.

After we complete the initial values assessment discovery, the next step in the design and development process is to begin to clarify how you can incorporate your core values into the daily activities that make up the bulk of your life! Remember, "My Life Well-Adjusted" is a process, not an event. I guarantee there may never be a process in your life that is more important or impactful!

Throughout this journey, you'll become more aware of your core values and begin to recognize how these character qualities interact with your life **vision, mission, and purpose**. As with anything worth doing, the end of the "My Life Well-Adjusted" process is really the beginning of the rest of your life. The 2-track system is designed to be a catalyst for action and a new found understanding to help guide you in the design of your ideal life in 7 dimensions (physical, mental, social, financial, spiritual, professional, and emotional).

Before you go any further in this chapter, and definitely before you decide to dig completely into this work, ask yourself the questions below, as they may help you realize if you're truly interested and/or definitely ready to begin designing and defining your life at this level.

1. Do I want to have a clearly designed and defined purposeful life and/or be one of the people my community turns to in times of need? If so, why? If not, why not?

_____

_____

_____

_____

_____

2. Am I willing or interested in investing the time, energy, and capital it takes to become the confident steward of my life purpose, and a valued and trusted person to others?

_____

_____

_____

_____

_____

3. Am I ready to start now?

_____!

I think I know the answer...let's get started!

Your purpose is the primary driver of true and lasting success. When you act without purpose, it leads to uncertainty, fear and eventually burnout, which will result in you getting stuck in the process. With a clearly defined purpose, the things you do have more meaning and lead to a more fulfilling outcome that is measurable against your vision.

When you define your purpose based on a series of values:

- You are able to see the true meaning of your actions and you are able to connect with your higher calling.

- You define your value or the worth of your actions and processes.

- You will have increased resolve, a higher sense of accomplishment, and accomplish more with less effort.

- You will have a more robust sense of self-esteem and realize deep rewards of greater personal and professional success.

Dr. Jeremy Book is a partner in the Chiropractic Vitality Centers of Maine, and the leader of Innate Family Chiropractic in South Portland, Maine. As a former professional athlete, he has a perspective most will never experience. Luckily for us, he shares his life experiences as a high-level athlete, honestly and openly, with our members and community. I've always pulled a lot from the article he shared in the "Wellness News You Can Use" newsletter called "Purpose."

Purpose

"Do you have a purpose in life? I hope you do. Having a purpose and passion for something in your life is one of the keys to longevity. If you have something to get excited and motivated about every day you drastically increase your odds of living a long and healthy life.

There are examples of this all around us. Think of the people you've known that seemed perfectly healthy, worked hard all their lives, and then their health went downhill after they retired. I see it all the time, life loses its luster when we lose our purpose. Or have you ever heard of someone who was terminally ill who continued to survive beyond all expectations because they had something that they needed to accomplish before they passed? This is very common and demonstrates the power of having purpose and passion in life.

In his book, "Man's Search for Meaning," Victor Frankle wrote that during his time in the concentration camps of World War II, he observed that the people who faired the best were those who were able to maintain hope of life beyond the camps. Some focused on their families, or some piece of important work they needed to accomplish. Those who lost all hope could not find anything inspiring to look forward to, they lost the will and the ability to cope with the harsh conditions of the concentration camps, and inevitably they were quick to perish.

Another great tip I once heard from a wise man was to connect your passion to your paycheck. Do you get excited about your work or do you trudge through the week counting down the hours to the weekend? I have been very fortunate to have 2 amazing careers, first as a professional pitcher for the St. Louis Cardinals organization, and now as a partner in the Chiropractic Vitality Centers of Maine. I have literally used my passion to provide for myself and my family for years. The activities you engage in every day will have a tremendous impact on your physical and mental health. So I would like to leave you with this quote below by Satchel Paige:

'Love like you have never been hurt, work like you don't need the money, and dance like no one is watching.'"

- Dr. Jeremy Book

To wrap up this brief overview of the values assessment process (trust me, this is a very brief overview of an in-depth discovery process), I invite you to begin working on your "purpose statement." I want to stress again that this process is usually completed over the course of multiple coaching sessions as well as time spent on your own, defining and refining this powerful statement. If you feel uncertain, confused, overwhelmed or uninspired, stop working on it now and schedule your initial consultation, as it's extraordinarily powerful when done with purpose!

What is your purpose statement? Why do you do the things you do? How are your values supported by your purpose, and how does your purpose support your values? Try to make it as complete and as short as possible. Also, there is no wrong statement.

_____

_____

_____

_____

_____

Your Vision Is your "What" (See Clearly)

Your **Vision** is the picture you create of what you want for yourself or for those you serve. It's the ultimate goal you hope to achieve as an outcome of your thoughts and actions. Your vision is a future tense construct. It's not in the here and now, it's an eventuality that you plan to see come to fruition, but you must see it as though it already exists.

Any successful venture, whether personal or professional, must be anchored with a vision of the outcome you desire to create. One of my mentors who radically helped me change my thoughts and actions in life is the late, and in my opinion great, Dr. Wayne Dyer. I'd like to share an idea that I picked up in my many hours of reading, listening to, and studying his life philosophies. My life was changed forever when I read these simple words in one of his books: "When you change the way you look at things, the things you look at change!" After I read that, I realized that I could create whatever I wanted in my life if I was willing to see challenging situations through a different lens or from a perspective that served me better. Not long afterward, I wrote and shared this article with our "Wellness News You Can Use" newsletter readers:

You'll See It When You Believe It!

"It's always interesting to see the reactions I get when I tell people "you'll see it when you believe it!" Often I get the quizzical stare of semi-awareness that they have heard something like that before, but it just doesn't sound or feel right in that order. That cognitive dissonance that happens is due to our familiarity with this similar phrase: "I'll believe it when I see it." The phrase we have all become accustomed to hearing is usually used in a very pessimistic or doubtful tone and with an energy that is rooted in helplessness or disbelief of possibilities. It is the ultimate phrase used to express the general lack of control most people feel they have in creating what they really want!

You see, we don't even realize it but over the years we have been conditioned to believe that what we want is only possible if we can witness it being done already. If we live life believing that we will only "believe it if we see it" then everything seems impossible unless it is proven possible by someone else. That is a very disempowered state! Creating the reality you want most is not a spectator sport, it is an ACTION SPORT!

The opposite of the usual term is the actual truth: "You will see it when you believe it." It is the power phrase that is at the heart of all success. "You will see it when you believe it" should really be adapted to all our lives and maybe even changed to "You will create it when you believe it!" This twist of the old fairytale myth of "waiting for something to happen" has the power to be an extreme catalyst for creation and is fuel to all endeavors that will lead to meaningful and fulfilling outcomes.

The proof of my thesis is the story of Roger Bannister, the first human to run a mile in under 4 minutes. Before he did that, no one had ever "seen" it done, so everyone except Roger thought it was impossible. In 1954, Roger was the only person that truly "believed" it was possible, and due to his belief in the possible, he proved to the world that it could be done. Since then, his record has been beat many times and now the record stands at an amazing 3:43:13, which is 17 seconds faster than the entire world believed could be done: that was until Roger Bannister knew it was possible.

It all starts with thought and/or belief! Do you believe you can be healthy, fit, free of pain, have abundant energy, age with grace and dignity, or any other amazing life feat? I believe you can and so do the doctors and teams at the Chiropractic Vitality Centers of Maine!"

What is your vision? The sky is the limit. What would your life look like if there were no rules and you could not fail? What would your multidimensional life look, feel, and act like as a result of your purposeful action? (The shorter the better. If you can answer this in 10 words or less, you are a superstar!)

_____

_____

_____

_____

_____

Our Mission is the "How" (Act Purposefully)

Your mission is a present time construct, it is the action, it is the "How." Your mission is your plan of purposeful action to accomplish the ultimate goal of seeing your vision materialize. When you have a well-defined mission statement, it helps you devise and implement strategies, coordinate patterns of actions, and accomplish outcomes that align with your values and vision. When you are on purpose it can seem like all the stars align and the opportunities to complete your task begin showing up effortlessly.

Not so fast though. If you're setting goals and achieving them, your vision and mission will most likely change as your personal and professional success grows. There is no end when you are on purpose, only new heights and higher aspirations.

When looking at life from a perspective of mission, we are really looking to define how we will think and act in the direction of the accomplishment of our goals and realization of our vision. To get our mission on an emotional and energetic level, beyond the ordinary daily chores or processes we engage in, we must begin to ask ourselves questions that help us define a deeper and more compelling purpose.

When we take life from the realm of processes to purpose, we take our journey from ordinary to extraordinary, and that ignites our creative juices and fans the flames of passion to dream and act bigger.

In the "My Life Well-Adjusted" curriculum, we focus on activities related to the 7 dimensions of our physical, mental, social, financial, spiritual, professional, and emotional lives, and in doing so we are able to develop a fully cohesive framework of success. The interesting result that comes from the focus on individual dimensions of life is that we begin to realize that in a fully developed and conscious life, there are no real defined borders between the 7 dimensions.

The process to purpose paradigm shift is such a powerful technique for focusing energy and attention that it becomes a framework that can guide life minute to minute or decade to decade. Imagine if your mission was so clear that you could easily decide what, where, and when to focus your attention and action throughout your day, week, month, or year! In the following article written by Dr. Mike Epperson, who leads our Richmond Family Chiropractic team in Richmond, Maine, he shares the concept of defining priorities and the power of staying on task.

Don't Give Up What You Want Most for What You Want Today

"I start each day with a focused planning session reviewing my expected accomplishments, it is my "power hour" (more like my power 10 minutes because it doesn't take an hour). I begin each day with the end-in-mind so I can plan my personal and professional life of purpose for the 24 hours I get that day. I am like everyone else, I have the same number of hours, the same number of tasks and obligations, and I have the same number of conflicting needs and desires. I realize that for me to be my best and to get the most out of my efforts I must stay focused on my ultimate mission, to be on purpose, not stuck in process. When I do this power hour, I create the direction necessary to coordinate my obligations to family, friends, patients, and coworkers in alignment with my purpose.

It can be challenging to keep the "plates spinning," but the rewards and sense of accomplishment at the end of the day make life what it is, an exciting, fun, and meaningful experience where we get to either step up to our greatness or shrink in defeat. I feel that planning my day is essential if I want to stay balanced and physically and emotionally healthy, but planning is not enough. I have found that I need to review my day continuously to stay on track and stay focused to avoid getting scattered and battered.

Each day of our lives we are given choices of how we show up. We are given crossroads to navigate and we are faced with decisions that not only affect our health and well-being in the moment, but shape our outcomes in the future. By reviewing throughout the day and recapping the day's events, attitudes, and actions, I can stay on track with immediate needs and long-term goals.

I have dedicated my adult years to serving people through the art, science, and philosophy of chiropractic, and what I have learned is this: When you give up what you want most for what you want in the moment it leads to one thing and one thing only, REGRET."

- Dr. Mike Epperson

When we have our core values as conscious directors of life, a clearly defined vision as a guide, and we engage in purposeful actions we can create the life that best serves us. If you want robust health, it takes persistent and consistent action supported by an unwavering commitment and discipline. If you want independent financial security, you must decide what is a long-term need and at times give up what you want now. This is a balancing act, as you want to make sure that you don't create a scarcity mentality around money, as that is not healthy either.

If what you want most in your relationships are for them to grow stronger, deeper, and more meaningful over time, it takes effort and planning. If what you want most is flexibility and physical freedom from injury and premature aging, don't wait, start today by consulting with a full-scope chiropractic practitioner to regain and maintain the structural, neurological, and physiological balance needed to achieve it.

If you feel you are going in the wrong direction professionally, start today by getting real clear on what you want and implement a purposeful plan to accomplish it. If you feel flat emotionally, spiritually, or mentally, now is the perfect time to dig into those areas of your life and define and design a new direction.

You are the author, creative director, and producer of your life. Just like a well-written, directed, and performed production, it takes time, effort, and rehearsal to get it right. To make sure you're creating a stirring and moving screenplay for life, make sure you have the vision set and begin to create the production of your dreams now!

As we did with the "Why" and "What", let's now work on the "How." In the space below, work on clarifying your mission. What is your mission? How will you accomplish your vision? This should be a statement of your plan to succeed. Hint: pick one aspect of your life in any of the 7 dimensions and use that as the subject of this initial statement.

It could be whatever is on your mind right now, such as a vision you have for your health, how you wish your relationship with your spouse to be, or what you plan to do for your kids as it pertains to college funding. There are literally countless areas that deserve this level of planning, and with each area you clarify, the other areas will become clearer as a result. As I suggested before, use the mind map technique to get it on paper then pare it down and define it into clarity.

_____

_____

_____

_____

_____

I know you're probably wondering what it takes to turn this chapter into reality in your life. Reading this and trying to implement these strategies alone, you may feel like it would be easier to drink water from a fire hydrant. Trust me, it's possible and worth the effort it takes to create your life on these terms. I'll reiterate what I said before, which is that I hesitated to include this chapter, as I didn't want to risk creating a sense of being overwhelmed for my readers.

This chapter is a brief overview and a generalized outline of a dedicated coaching and care program directed as an intensive one on one, 52-week life adjustment program. So please don't feel overwhelmed or discount the idea that you can accomplish everything I've laid out, and more! You can create the life you want most, you have everything you need to succeed, you deserve to have a well-defined and designed life, and it is worth the effort!

Thank you for taking this literary journey with me. I now invite you to take a literal journey to your well-adjusted life if you're ready. I love the direction my years of experience have taken me, and I strive to help my clients develop a life that is truly rewarding and fulfilling in all dimensions.

Co-founding the 5 offices that make up the Chiropractic Vitality Centers of Maine and sharing my experience with my fellow partners has been a dream come true! Seeing our practice members and communities thrive with full-scope chiropractic care has been one of my greatest passions, and I'm proud to continue my career with Bangor Family Chiropractic. Adding the strength of the "My Life Well-Adjusted" program to the structural, neurological, and physiological balance of full-scope chiropractic care has taken the results of my early work to an entirely new dimension. I'm excited to share it with you!

"Who We Be" determines "What We Create."

Chapter 10

The 7 Dimensions of Life

This chapter is dedicated to Dr. Alan Rousso who has been my coach, friend, and mentor. Without his patience, guidance, and support, this book would not have been possible.

When life is in balance in all dimensions, everything works as it should and every aspect of life contributes and enhances the whole. The converse is also true. When our lives are out of balance in any dimension it will ultimately diminish or detract from the quality of the whole. Being out of balance affects our energy, stamina, creativity, drive, and determination. With imbalance comes ineffective or limited thoughts and actions, and therefore limited outcomes. If you want to get the most out of life, you must maximize every dimension of life. When that happens, you'll be amazed at the freedom it creates!

When "My Life Well-Adjusted" clients start their journey, it becomes very clear to them where their biggest obstacles are, and in which dimension or dimensions they are having the most interference. For some, it comes from their thoughts: "I can't do that," "I've never been the kind of person who…," "If I try that and fail I will be disappointed," etc.

Sometimes the interference comes from deeply held beliefs related to our upbringing, and how we were influenced by our mother, father, teacher, preacher, or others. Sometimes it comes from a fear of loss or failure. Regardless of the origin of the obstacles, the uncertainty and hesitation they breed causes interference in the movement of life through wrong actions or inaction. In the end, the totality of your life today is the accumulation of your thoughts, your beliefs, and your actions!

There is no shortcut to the ideal life, but there is a roadmap with very specific directions and really cool attractions along the way. Imagine feeling fully empowered by your thoughts. Can you picture a world where you believe you can accomplish any goal? It sounds intriguing and inspiring, doesn't it?

Can you picture yourself being the perfect weight? Do you desire to have a more abundant supply or cushion of money? Would you love to have great relationships in your life? Do you ever feel the pressure of taking on too much, and wish you had more free time? How about waking up each morning feeling energized and ending the day fully charged? You deserve to live a life knowing that your physical health is improving daily, weekly, monthly, and that someday you will be able to fully enjoy a time where you have everything you want and need, and you are prepared to retire and PLAY!

A Well-Adjusted Life is Balanced in 7 Key Areas

The goal of *beginning* the "My Life Well-Adjusted" process is to *end* with a well-defined and well-designed life that is the reflection of your desires, and a life you know you deserve. Life is a journey with many destinations and it should be lived with as much vitality, imagination, definition, and verve as possible.

Living a well-adjusted life means living a life of conscious awareness. It means that you have a self-

146

determined "Why", a clearly defined "What", and a well-designed "How." When we combine the 2 tracks of full-scope chiropractic and whole life planning and development, we create the possibilities of an inspired and meaningful outcome that most people only dream about, but everyone deserves.

My goal in practicing the "My Life Well-Adjusted" model is to take my members through a process of creating the possibility of living the richest and most rewarding life possible. I've seen different levels of success with the members I've worked with. Some focus more on one or 2 specific dimensions, and some focus on all of them. The key is this: wherever your attention goes, your energy flows!

The life you ultimately build will be a result of the energy and focus you put into it. There are no guarantees in life, of course, other than death and taxes. But there are reasons to work hard to create possibilities that are amazing! In the early chapters, I covered (in detail) the reasons to incorporate full-scope chiropractic care into your life. For the remainder of this chapter, I'll explain the expected outcomes of the whole life planning and development phase of track 2 of "My Life Well-Adjusted."

Phase 1: Physical Balance

In phase 1, we will primarily focus on getting your physical life in balance. This will begin with the initial consultation, examination, optimal care recommendations, and the successful progression of a 3-phase program of full-scope chiropractic care. Your full-scope chiropractic care program will focus on spinal and neurological adjustments to maximize your body's ability to self-regulate, regain and maintain a maximal adaptive state, and ensure you can meet the physical, mental/emotional, and chemical stress of life successfully.

The measurements we will use include: postural screening, nervous system assessments, full spine x-ray evaluation, physical activity and range of motion measurements, body mass index, weight, 7-point body measurements, and a physiological test to analyze where you are off nutritionally. This phase, starting day 1 and extending for a full year will help you achieve the following goals and more:

1) Reduce the progression and/or eliminate the development of arthritis.

2) Develop a strong and balanced spinal system and coordinated muscular system.

3) Maximize the ability of your brain and body to communicate and increase your ability to self-regulate and achieve optimal health expression.

4) Regain and maintain the ideal weight, build habits around food and hydration that will create the foundation for life, build a rock-solid metabolism, and become confident in your lifestyle.

5) Design and implement a custom flexibility program and exercise plan to help you hit your target goals of strength, endurance, stamina, and agility.

6) Build a consistent workout plan that you can do anywhere, anytime, without the need of expensive equipment or gym memberships.

7) Reduce and/or eliminate the need for drugs, the likelihood of injury, and your risk of diabetes, heart disease, cancer, stroke, and all other lifestyle-related disorders.

The Physical Balance phase continues through the course of the entire 52-week program.

Phase 2: Mental, Emotional, Spiritual Balance

In phase 2, we support the physical manifestation of health achieved in phase 1 with the design and development of daily, weekly, monthly, and lifelong habits of thought. Once you begin to function better physically we want to add a layer of living better in the mental, emotional, and spiritual realms.

This phase is where we begin to build your mental strength and agility using, among other things, books, audios, movies, empowering stories of others, visualization, vision boarding, goal setting, and behaviors that reinforce the balance built in both phase 1 and 2.

Phase 2, starting at the end of phase 1 and continuing through the remainder of the 52-week program will help you achieve the following goals, activities, beliefs, and behaviors:

1) A healthy and empowered self-image.

2) The understanding of the power of visualizing success and looking for the outcomes that reinforce your goals.

3) You will define your ideal life in all 7 dimensions with the help of a vision board and daily affirmations.

4) You will define your ideal spiritual anchor/anchors and use them in your daily life as inspiration and strength.

5) You will learn to love learning again and will become fascinated with the world inside and around you.

6) You will learn to view the world through the eyes of positive probabilities and learn to quiet thoughts of negative possibilities.

7) You will use the power of your new mental, emotional, spiritual habits in the form of volunteerism and/or mentorship in your community. (Community may mean a one-on-one relationship with a friend or family member or a group of individuals).

8) You will believe in yourself enough to set an audacious goal, start a new project, finish a previously scrapped effort, tackle any previously perceived weaknesses, and stay disciplined to accomplish what you start!

If any of this gives you jitters, that may be the best reason ever to start your journey.

Phase 3: Professional, Social, Financial Balance

For many, the 3 dimensions of phase 3 are the most ill-defined and under-designed aspect of life. In the "My Life Well-Adjusted" model, we understand that life can be a beautiful quilt of interwoven dimensions that work in harmony and balance, or it can end up being a tattered patchwork of ill-fitting dimensions and frayed edges.

In the final (not absolute, the journey starts here for some) phase of the journey, we'll focus on who you BE at work, at home, in your community, and in your financial world. The wholeness of your experience in life is reconciled, in part, by the quality and the quantity of the relationships you have at work, in your personal life, and in your financial world.

The culmination of the work of phase 3 is to ensure that these dimensions are in coordination and not competition with each other. Phase 3 as a continuation of phase 2, and as the culmination of the 52-week program will help you achieve the following goals, activities, beliefs, and behaviors:

1) Define your ideal professional life including position, profession, path, and vision.

2) Define and design the who, what, and when of your social life.

3) Set targeted and achievable goals for your financial life.

You will be able to see how these 3 dimensions of life feed and nurture each other.

If you should decide to use this as a starting point on a life long journey of discovery and empowerment, congratulations! If you decide that you want to build your well-adjusted life using this book as a guide map, I hope you succeed beyond your wildest dreams! If you've decided that you want to work with me to coach, facilitate, challenge, and celebrate you on your journey to your well-adjusted life, I am ready!

It has been a difficult task to take this work from practice to print, but it has been worth it, and it's a reflection of many of the dimensions of my well-adjusted life.

Thank you for taking the time to read "My Life Well-Adjusted!" It is my biggest hope that it serves you well! To end this chapter, conclude the body of this book, and to help you start a journey to your well-adjusted life, I will leave you with a simple but powerful exercise. Please ponder this question for each of the 7 dimensions of your well-adjusted life.

What's one thing you could change, or an inspired goal that would make the biggest impact in each area of your well-adjusted life?

Physical:

_____

_____

_____

Mental

_____

_____

_____

Social

_____

_____

_____

Financial

_____

_____

_____

Spiritual

_____

_____

_____

Professional

_____

_____

_____

Emotional

_____

_____

_____

If there is one thing that you know would be the biggest obstacle to your making any or all of these changes, what would it be?

_____

_____

_____

_____

_____

How important do you feel coaching and accountability will be to you in building the foundation for the life you desire and deserve?

1   2   3   4   5   6   7   8   9   10

To schedule a consult with Dr. Jeffrey Slocum you can do so by using this information:

Dr. Jeffrey Slocum, owner of Bangor Family Chiropractic and developer and head coach at My Life Well-Adjusted
207-307-7513 • drjeff@mylifewelladjusted.com

Terms

Vertebral Subluxation Complex: When we add "complex" to the vertebral subluxation we do so to define the five distinct component that combine to create a spinal or vertebral subluxation complex. These five are:

1. The Osseous Component is where the vertebra are either out of position, not moving properly or are undergoing physical changes such as degeneration. This component is sometimes known as vertebral subluxation.

2. The Nerve Component is the malfunctioning nerve. Research has shown that only a small amount of pressure on the spinal nerves can have a profound impact on the function of nerves. This component is scientifically known as neuropathology.

3. The Muscle Component is also involved. Since muscles help hold the vertebrae in place, and since nerves control the muscles themselves, muscles are an integral part of any VSC. In fact, muscles both affect, and are affected by the VSC. This component is known as myopathology.

4. The Soft Tissue Component is when there are misaligned vertebrae and the pressure on nerves resulting in changes to the surrounding soft tissues. This means the tendons, ligaments, blood supply, and other tissues undergo changes. These changes can occur at the point of the VSC or far away at

some end point of the affected nerves. This component is known as histopathology.

5. The Chemical Component is when all of these components of the VSC are acting on your body, and therefore causing some degree of chemical changes. Theses chemical changes can be slight or massive depending on what parts of the body are affected by your subluxations. This component is often known as biochemical abnormalities. *Dr. Christopher Raymond*

Homeostasis: The tendency of the body to seek and maintain a condition of balance or equilibrium within its internal environment, even when faced with external changes. A simple example of homeostasis is the body's ability to maintain an internal temperature around 98.6 degrees Fahrenheit, whatever the temperature outside.

Motor Nervous System: Sensory/afferent neurons carry the impulses from the body to the central nervous system and the brain. After being processed by the central nervous system, the somatic motor, or efferent, neurons take the signal back to the muscles and sensory organs. Afferent and Efferent Neurons.

Somatic Nervous System: The autonomic nervous system has 2 divisions: the sympathetic nervous system, which accelerates the heart rate, constricts blood vessels, and raises blood pressure, and the parasympathetic nervous system, which slows the heart rate, increases intestinal and gland activity, and relaxes sphincter muscles.

Symptomatic: Being a symptom of a disease. b : having the characteristics of a particular disease but arising from another cause.

Asymptomatic: If you're asymptomatic, you don't show any signs of being sick. In some cases, you can have a disease but still be asymptomatic.

Mechanoreceptor: We and other animals have several types of receptors of mechanical stimuli. Each initiates nerve impulses in sensory neurons when it is physically deformed by an outside force such as: touch; pressure; stretching; sound waves; motion

Nociceptor: A receptor for pain, stimulated by various kinds of tissue injury. ... A peripheral nerve organ or mechanism for the reception and transmission of painful or injurious stimuli. ... a somatic and visceral free nerve ending of thinly myelinated and unmyelinated fibers.

Somatic: relating to the wall of the body cavity, especially as distinguished from the head, limbs, or viscera. 3. Of or relating to the portion of the vertebrate nervous system that regulates voluntary movement.

Visceral: Referring to the viscera, the internal organs of the body, specifically those within the chest (as the heart or lungs) or abdomen (as the liver, pancreas or intestines). In a figurative sense, something "visceral" is felt "deep down." It is a "gut feeling."

Research

Measurable changes within the joint complex occur within one week of the onset of hypo mobility.

Lantz C., Immobilization degeneration and the fixation hypothesis of chiropractic subluxation. Chiro Research Journal; 1988;1(1):21-45

Preexisting connective tissue trauma increases immobilization; Any patient with a history of spinal injury should be evaluated for biomechanical instability, symptomatic or not. *Marwah. International Orthopedics, 1985. Burks, et al. Am J of Sports Medicine, 1984.*

The disc lives because of movement. Hypomobility causes decreased hydraulic action on the disc, therefore decreasing the ability of the disc to gain essential nutrients, blood, and water, as well as eliminate waste. The inner portion of the disc, the nucleus pulposus, is avascular. The effect of hypo mobility in the synthesis of degenerative arthritis causes the uptake of calcium blocking the bony channels of nutrient flow to the nucleus. *Mooney, Spine, 1987*

Neurological Effects of Hypo mobility: In the presence of a vertebral subluxation complex the sympathetic nervous system is recruited and facilitated through synaptic activity of the spinal cord. *Lisa Bloom DC, DACS, DIBCN*

The dorsal horn is a central focal point for mediating autonomic and somatomotor reflexes initiated by nociceptive stimulation. Sensitization of spinal cord neurons primarily by C fibers from muscles, joints, and periosteum causes prolonged increased excitability of the cells. *D. Psychological and Neural Mechanisms of Pain, 1988; Raven Press, NY.*

Vertebral subluxation complex results in: altered somatic function, altered visceral function, allodynia, sustained pain syndromes. *Bonica JJ. Clinical importance of hyperalgesia in hyeralgesia and allodynia; WD Willis Jr.,ed. Raven Press, Ltd., NY; 17-43.*

Nociceptor activity reflexively activates the sympathetic nervous system. Noxious chemical stimulation of specific spinal structures produce measurable changes in sympathetic nerve activity and visceral function. Budgell B, et al. Spinovisceral reflexes evoked by noxious and innocuous stimulation of the lumbar spine. *J Neuromuskuloskeletal Syst; 1995;3:122-131. The Effects of Nociceptive Activity: Segmental responses of muscle spasm and sympathetic hyperactivity J. Bonica, 1990 & 1992, Hooshmand, 1993.*

Stimulation of sympathetic preganglionic neurons results in: increased cardiac work, increased myocardial oxygen consumption. If severe enough, may cause arrhythmia, decreased gastrointestinal tone, decreased tone of urinary track. *Lisa Bloom DC, DACS, DIBCN*

Structures receiving direct innervation by the sympathetic nervous system: blood vessels, intervertebral discs, mucous linings, bone marrow, hair follicles, sweat glands, arteries, endocrine system (adrenal gland sympathetic nervous system only), immune system organs, digestive, cardiovascular, pulmonary systems, mast cells, & gonads, ocular reflex muscles.

The visceral effects of vertebral subluxation complex: Dr. Windsor studied several hundred human and feline cadavers in 1921 at the University of Pennsylvania and found a correlation between organ disease and spinal misalignment in nearly 100% of the diseased cadavers. *The Windsor Autopsies*

Headaches: "It appears that chiropractors have been right all along. A team of doctors at Syracuse University have established with scientific, anatomical proof, that damaged structures (subluxations) are the cause of many chronic headaches." *Dec. 28, 1995. Life Toronto Star: Life section Peter Rothbart M.D.*

Spinal Learning (Law of Facilitation): Altered motor and sensory patterns are "learned" by the nervous system and the musculoskeletal systems. Repeated/chronic firing along a neural sequence results in a lowering of the electrical resistance along that pathway. *Lisa Bloom DC, DACS, DIBCN*

161

Bio-mechanical Effects of Subluxation:

- Altered intersegmental movement patterns
- Results in compensatory changes in motor patterns, etc.
- Creates cellular damage in sites of biomechanical stresses

Immobilization Degeneration

- Altered Biomechanics/Decreased mechanoreceptor activity
- Breaking of cells and release of irritants histamine, lactic acid, and bradykinin
- Firing of spinal chemosensitive nociceptors which now lack the inhibitory effect of the normal mechanoreceptor activation
- Which leads to increased sympathetic nervous system activity

Proper Assessment of vertebral subluxation complex:

- Must include a thorough history including childhood trauma
- Must include postural assessment visual inspection seated, standing, and prone
- Must include both static and motion palpation of the spine and surrounding tissue
- Must incorporate testing to assess motor and autonomic nervous system function
- Probable inclusion of x-ray analysis to visualize degree of degenerative changes to help assess length of instability and severity of progression

About the Author

Dr. Jeffrey Slocum is a 1993 graduate of Logan College in St. Louis, Missouri and has been in private practice full-time for 25 years. He is a 4th generation chiropractor and the 11th member of his family to practice chiropractic.

Dr. Slocum is the founder of the Chiropractic Vitality Centers of Maine and owner of Slocum Chiropractic "A Creating Wellness Center" in Brunswick, Maine, Richmond Family Chiropractic in Richmond, Maine, Innate Family Chiropractic in S. Portland, Maine, and Bangor Family Chiropractic in Bangor, Maine.

Dr. Slocum is a co-creator of Learning Curves™ and The Legion of Chiropractic and hosts an annual seminar in Mexico called Purposeful Connections. He is the developer of a highly successful personal and professional training company called Advanced Leadership Solutions.

Together he and his partners provide the most dynamic leadership development programs in the chiropractic profession. Dr. Slocum lectures nationally and internationally to chiropractors, encouraging them to spread awareness of chiropractic in their communities.

Dr. Jeff as he is known has been featured as the keynote speaker for the Maine Municipal Association's annual conventions, where he has helped thousands of municipal employees gain access to chiropractic coverage in Maine.

Dr. Slocum was named one of the most influential chiropractors under 40 by Chiropractic Lifestyles magazine in 2008. He was featured as the On Purpose Chiropractor of the Month in July, 2008, as well as being awarded the 2004 Chiropractor of the Year for The Masters Circle. He has spoken to the Student WCA, The American Chiropractor conference in Panama, New Beginnings, Bath Iron Works (a division of General Dynamics Corp.) and many other groups and organizations including state Boards of Education.

Dr. Slocum is regularly heard on Brican's Path To Excellence, and been a contributor for The American Chiropractor magazine.

Visit bangorfamilychiropractic.com to schedule your full-scope chiropractic consult or e-mail at drjeff@bangorfamilychiropractic.com or call (207) 307-7513 to schedule your My Life Well-Adjusted consultation or to have Dr. Slocum speak at your next event.

Made in the USA
Thornton, CO
10/14/22 12:07:01

13d09adb-7edc-44d8-ac4d-fa5adc718e72R01